Life Unexpected

A Trauma Psychologist Journeys Through Breast Cancer

Naomi L. Baum

Naomi L. Baum
POB 1159
Efrat, Israel   90435
www.naomibaum.com

Book Layout ©2013 BookDesignTemplates.com

Cover Art: " Tree of Life " by Ricardo Lowenberg used with permission of artist.

Ordering Information:
Quantity sales. Special discounts are available on quantity purchases by corporations, associations, and others. For details, contact Naomi.baum@gmail.com.

Life Unexpected: A Trauma Psychologist Journeys through Breast Cancer/ Naomi L. Baum. —1st ed.
ISBN 978-1499532920

Contents

*This book is dedicated
to my family,
whose love and support never wavered.*

Foreward:

Tenth Anniversary Edition

I am sitting looking out on a bucolic scene in upstate NY.

Rolling green fields, a weathered barn that is our home for a week, dogs barking, hens cackling, a tractor firing up, and lots of silence. This is the perfect time to write an introduction to the tenth anniversary edition of "Life Unexpected: A Trauma Psychologist Journeys Through Breast Cancer," a book that I published back in 2014. Sitting here I realized that my cancer diagnosis was exactly 12 years ago, almost to the day! I finished treatments- surgery, chemo, and radiation more than eleven years ago.

What has happened in the interim? How have I picked up the pieces to my life? What has changed and what has stayed the same? What wisdom can I share that will help fellow sojourners on the road to recovery and health? Is this book still relevant? Still helpful? All these questions and more flood my brain.

So I'll start from the end. I believe this book is a true account of my journey, and many people may find that it resonates with some or most of their experiences. If there is one thing that I have learned from my cancer journey it is that each and every one of us are unique. What works for one person, doesn't necessarily work for the other. That goes for chemo, medications, alternative or complementary therapies, diets, and more. If you find this book helpful, wonderful! If you find yourself arguing and dismissing every other word, let it go! You don't have to finish the book. It is certainly not the gospel truth. It is simply my take on my very personal and particular journey with breast cancer.

In the past six years I have been most fortunate to partner with an organization in Israel, Revadim, that runs retreats based on the "Commonweal" model, helping women who are on the healing journey. I have been blessed to meet many women from all walks of life, ages, types of cancers and degrees of illness, all bravely looking this disease in the eye, and taking a pause to consider where they are in their own lives. This experience has further confirmed for me how many roads there are to walk on this cancer journey.

If I look back at the curves in my road, cancer was certainly a big one. It gave me pause. It actually did more than that. It stopped me clear in my tracks and said, where are you going? What are you doing? And perhaps most importantly, what do you want to do now?

Since completing cancer treatment there are many parts of my life that have picked up and continued, and there are others that changed radically. My husband, children, and extended family have remained the core, the very heart of my existence. Professionally I exited my leadership position at the leading trauma center in Jerusalem and continued as an independent consultant and freelancer in the field, picking and choosing the work I wanted to do, and deciding how much and when I wanted to do it. Freeing up so much time allowed me to write several books, spend more time with grandchildren and children, travel, volunteer, and teach Qigong.

This introduction has also allowed me to consider what was missing in the original book. Revisiting the long process of healing from cancer treatment, I have come to realize that while much focus is placed on the actual treatment phase, once it is concluded we are expected to quickly and easily return to the way "we used to be." Most people around us have used up their patience and understanding during that long year of treatment. They are ready for us to pick up the reins and bounce back.

This of course is true if we are lucky enough to reach remission or shift to a chronic and more minor player on the stage of life.

In talking with many people who have undergone cancer treatment, the period of time after active treatment has concluded may be the most difficult to navigate. The expectation that "I am all better", and the fantasy that life will return to the way it used to be, is often severely shattered.

I think that a closer examination of the concept of resilience may help us here. My understanding of resilience is that bouncing back to the way we used to be is NOT the key. Rather, considering the notion of bouncing forward nay be more helpful. It is a truism to state that we will never return to be the people we were before that earthquake called cancer. We are different. We feel different. Cancer has changed us and shaped us. For many of us the change is very palpable and physical. For most of us it is both spiritual and emotional. Some may feel scarred, others feel frightened. Yet others may feel empowered. There is not one single trajectory of growth and recovery that is true for all who had cancer. But one thing I know for certain. This "post treatment" phase should be acknowledged and recognized both by ourselves and by those who surround us, love us and support us. Acknowledging the unique qualities of this period of time may allow us to be more patient with ourselves, and help us explain ourselves to the people around us.

As I look back on the more than a decade after completing cancer treatment, if someone were to ask me what are the keys to recovering from cancer and living the good life, I would boil it down to five:

1. *Don't push things off for a later date. If you want to visit the Taj Mahal or Timbuktu, get online and make your reservations today. We never know what is around the corner, and as wise cancer survivors, we know that there is no time like the present.*

2. *Tell your children and spouse that you love them. Of course they know that you love them, but tell them. Tell them! Tell them today! And tell them often!*

3. *Become proactive with your physical self. Invite into your life the things that make you feel good and that you enjoy. Whether it be a vegetarian lifestyle, cycling, walking, meditating, pushups, yoga, Qigong, none of the above, or all of the above, make sure that you move, and make sure that whatever you choose, you do it with joy.*

4. **Surround yourself with people that you love. Cancer often helps us separate the wheat from the chaff on many levels. One of those is friendships. Make sure to invest in the friends that are dear to you. The others, you can let go.**

5. **Ask yourself, what else do you want to do with your life? What gives your life meaning? What gives you a good reason to wake up in the morning? If you aren't sure, and sometimes that happens after healing from cancer, give yourself some time, but don't forget the question. This is a seminal question that you must address, sooner or later. Better sooner.**

One of the things that has struck me in my work with women who are healing from cancer is the fear factor. Learning to live with the fear of recurrent cancer is a fact of life that is not often discussed openly. In Chapter 14 of this book you will find an entire chapter about fear, yet after more than ten years, I'd like to share with you that fear of recurrence does not disappear. It does not dissolve. In my experience, we will never return to being the carefree people we were before having cancer. The niggling fear that cancer will return is never far from our consciousness if we are honest with ourselves. What to do about it? Read bullet points 1-5 above. I think that is the answer, at least for me. That is what I do about the fear. Fear can paralyze all of us if we let it. The key for me is to acknowledge its presence, and then go on and live as if it is not there.

Several months ago we lost our dear son, Didi, to cancer. He left this earth in a chariot of fire, like Elijah the prophet, without warning, without preparation. He discovered a large tumor, and underwent aggressive surgery from which he never returned. His journey into cancer was so different from mine, that it feels like an entirely different disease. This reminds me to be modest in all of my pronouncements. What I speak about in this book, I speak simply from my experience, which is that of one woman who discovered that she had breast cancer, and what happened next. Nothing, but nothing has prepared me for dealing with the terrible loss of a son, yet it occurs to me that those five bullet points above have kept me going through these long dark months of mourning as well. We can't always do each one of those five keys to resilience at once. Sometimes we need to sit quietly, and be gentle with ourselves, allowing ourselves time to heal. Yet, knowing that the day will come when we will once again take on the world, each in our own unique way, to lead our best lives, is a healing thought.

Sending blessings of health and healing,

Naomi Baum, June 2023

Prologue

Beginning at the end, I am starting to write this book in Venice, city of faded glories and opulent past. This is a celebration trip. A celebration of life. A celebration of completing nearly a year of cancer treatments and coming out on the other end.

On the very last day of my last radiation treatment, as my steadfast walking partner and I began our daily paces, I noted that it was almost exactly nine months since I was diagnosed with breast cancer. She asked me, without missing a beat, "So what have you given birth to?" The question startled me for a moment and then took hold. I had been talking for a couple of years about writing a book, and all of a sudden it became clear to me that this was the book: Surviving Breast Cancer - Mind, Body and Soul. And so the idea for the book was born. Now it remains for me to complete it.

My journey into breast cancer began as unexpectedly as it ever does. No family history, no particular worries about breast cancer had crossed my horizon. As another friend whose daughter survived cancer told me, it's always the things you least expect that show up on your screen. Cancer caught me one   fine   sunny   day,   totally   by surprise.

This book is a gift to you, a travel guide of sorts to accompany you through the foreign terrain and customs you may encounter in your odyssey through the land of cancer. I will share with you – whether you be patient, survivor, family member or friend – some of what I have learned on my personal journey.

I bring to this book both my personal experiences, as well as my professional expertise as a psychologist who specializes in the field of trauma. Resilience building has informed my professional life for the past decade (see Appendix), and in the past year it has served as the anchor and beacon in my personal life, as I traveled the path of breast cancer. I have developed resilience building programs for educators, first responders and other communities touched by trauma over these last many years at my professional home, the Israel Center for the Treatment of Psychotrauma in Jerusalem. I started off this year knowing a lot about trauma and resilience, and having met many people whose lives had been touched, shattered, or battered by trauma, and from whom I had learned and been inspired. However, I humbly submit that this year was the greatest teacher of all. I hope to share with you some of what I have learned.

My personal experiences that form the backdrop to this story,
include the fact that I have been married for well over three decades to the same wonderful human being. Mike and I have raised seven children (yup-seven) and have become enthusiastic grandparents to a gaggle of grandchildren. We moved to Israel from the United States a quarter of a century ago and make our home near Jerusalem.Both my professional and my personal lives have informed this book as they directed me in my quest. One of the understandings I have come to over

the years is how mind, body and spirit are all connected and the essence of what makes us human. Cancer is a physical disease and as such, the focus of cancer care is often primarily the physical body. Much time is spent going from test to test, physician to physician, and treatment to treatment. The "body" part of cancer is undeniable and is addressed by many others in books, magazine
articles and online. The parts of cancer that are often overlooked, however, are the mind and spirit. In recent years, many of us have learned and re-learned that these are key to recovery. In this book, as I share with you my healing journey, I will consider these three elements that are, to my mind, crucial to recovery: mind, body and spirit.

A word about terms is in order here: Patients? Sufferers? Survivors? What shall we call ourselves? Each word conveys a distinct aspect of the experience, relevant at a different point in time. Every time I try to put a name to what I am, I end up mumbling something or other, and then end with, "I was treated for cancer." That is objective, undeniable, and true. So the various terms listed above are used interchangeably in the text, and if they don't suit you, feel free to mentally switch any one of them for whatever word feels best to you.

Another semantic note, that is far more than just words. I use the term "healing journey" throughout this book. My travels through cancer became a healing journey almost from the moment I was
diagnosed with that life-threatening disease.It was clear to me from that moment onwards I would do my utmost to heal myself as best I could in order to continue living a productive,

meaningful life. My focus on healing took many forms over the course of the year, which I hope to share with you. First and foremost was the proactive
decision to feel that even though I had not chosen to have cancer, and it was something that happened to me,
nevertheless I would take back as much control over my life as I could. Clearly, making the
decision to focus on healing and life is simpler if you are not suffering from physical symptoms that cause weakness and pain. Luckily, I was still feeling fine. But no matter how you are feeling, to my mind, it is an absolutely essential decision to make if we are to have a fighting chance in overcoming this disease and returning to health and life. I urge you to join me in that focus on healing and health as we embark together on this journey to."

[1]

Diagnosis: D-Day

Our long anticipated, one-month vacation was on the horizon. The June sun was shining with not a cloud in the sky. There was nothing to augur what an eventful day this was to be in my life. I went about my business with no premonitions, no butterflies in my stomach, and no worries, other than getting my life organized before setting out to the airport with my husband in a week's time. I was tying up loose ends at work, cleaning out the fridge, beginning to pack, and to say goodbye to friends.

Picture the scene: It is early afternoon and I am at work. I am consulting with psychologists in a rural Bedouin town in the south of Israel, about an hour's drive from Jerusalem. Women of all sizes and shapes are swishing by wearing long coats, their faces entirely swathed in scarves. Swarthy, lean men in black and red kaffiyas, the traditional Bedouin headgear, abound. I am sitting in a sparsely furnished office with a local psychologist who works with me. We are discussing the fine points of facilitating resilience-building groups. These groups train teachers to help their students deal with trauma. Over the course of the group sessions we teach the teachers about how trauma affects us all, how teachers can help themselves and how they can then bring that knowledge and skill base to their classrooms. I am supervising the psychologist's work with a recent group of teachers.

My cell phone rings. I usually don't take calls during work, but the screen flashes with my husband's name and as he does not usually call me, I think it might be urgent and decide to answer. I excuse myself and take the call. My husband, not sounding at all like himself says,

"Hi Naomi. How are you?" My usually busy husband sounds like he has all the time in the world.

"What's up?" I quickly ask. My heartbeat intuitively speeds up

before my mind can even catch up.

"The results came back from your biopsy and it's not good." Mike says abruptly.

"What? How could that be?" I practically shout into the phone, not paying attention to the psychologist sitting nearby.

I had had a mammogram and ultrasound the week before that were both clear. The doctor, as part of the physical exam, had

palpated a lymph node in my right underarm that he thought seemed bigger than it should have been, and he biopsied it just to make sure all was okay. He told me that in the last four years only one sample that he had biopsied had been positive. Guess who was the second?

The results came directly through to my husband, a physician, since I had listed him as the referring physician. To this day I don't really know how he reacted upon receiving the results. I do know that it took him several hours to call me, and that when he did finally make the call, he did not sound like himself at all. I wonder, too, why he didn't ask me where I was, and who was with me. He just blurted out the results as if he could hold them in no longer.

My immediate response to the news was, "this can't be true." My husband opened the file and read the results to me twice, so I could take it all in. From the moment he started reading I became extremely present and aware. I could feel every muscle and bone in my body. I can recall exactly where I sat, what the room looked like, what time of day it was, and how quickly my heart was beating. Everything was in sharp relief, an almost out-of-body experience. As I write this almost a year later, I can still picture the scene in exquisite detail.

Since my conversation with my husband had been in English, the psychologist I had been meeting with did not follow it, and after closing the phone, I quickly tried to pick up the meeting where we had left off, as if my world had not just collapsed on me. It took me only a few minutes, during which thoughts raced through my head at breakneck speed, to realize that I needed to end the meeting immediately. The surprised psychologist whom I had come to supervise said goodbye and I beat a hasty retreat. I just barely made it to my car before the tears started rolling down my cheeks. Without waiting a moment to catch my breath, I started the car and began my ride homeward.

I remember that hour-long drive back to Jerusalem vividly. Corny as it sounds now, my life passed before my eyes, as if on a movie screen. I thought about all the blessings in my life – my seven children, my husband, parents, brothers, sister, and extended family. I thought about how fortunate I had been to have both a rich personal and professional life. I remembered vacations, hikes and holidays, and thought about close friends. All of this in the course of one hour: "My life – the Condensed Version." While the tears slowly coursed down my cheeks, I was overwhelmed by feelings of both thankfulness and loss. Thankfulness for what I had been the beneficiary of until now; loss for what I might be missing in the future – children's marriages, births of grandchildren, great-grandchildren and more. I pictured many of these events without me, in great detail, and tears just continued to roll down my face as the kilometers peeled away. And then I looped back again to gratefulness, thankful for my fifty-six full years.

As the road wound up the hills to Jerusalem, a new thought entered my mind. "This is the beginning of a journey." I had a strong, almost physical, sense that this cancer was divinely driven. Now, if only I could figure out the purpose of this disease, why I got it, and what I was supposed to make of it, I might have a direction.

These two attitudes – gratefulness and an appreciation of the
divinely-driven nature of the cancer – and for that matter- my life, announced themselves in the very first hour after the diagnosis. They have continued to accompany me along my entire   odyssey.   My feelings of loss and mourning certainly did not disappear completely, but rather gradually receded over the next several weeks as I made a very conscious decision not to wallow in feelings of "poor me" or "why me?" I knew now, more than ever before, that my time on this earth was limited. I had a choice: I could live it mindfully, with joy and gratitude or I could feel sorry for myself, mourn my lost health, my lost opportunities, and all the "could haves" and "should haves." The choice was an easy one for me.

Gratitude and recognition of a higher power have guided this journey from the start. My feelings of gratefulness for all the support and love from family and friends have only grown. Regarding the divinely-driven nature of the illness, I wish that I could say, "I now know exactly why I got cancer and what the divine

purpose in it was." Unfortunately, I cannot do that. I certainly have considered this long and hard and will share with you some of my best guesses, as well as some wise thoughts that others have shared with me along the way.

In the early days of my breast cancer, I woke up each morning to a visual image of a larger-than-life poster flashing before my eyes in bright red capital letters spelling out **"BREAST CANCER"**. This image descended upon me even before I had opened my eyes. It was my first thought upon waking and my last thought before falling asleep. In those early days, I was very caught up in the whys, the wherefores, and the lessons to be learned and appreciated. I searched my lifestyle, my health habits, my gene pool, my diet, and came up with small hints, but no overarching reason why I, of all people, should be diagnosed with breast cancer. Some clues included having a family history of various types of cancers (not breast). In addition, I have led a fairly intense life over the last thirty years, raising a family of seven children, and pursuing a demanding career in the field of trauma psychology. Regarding environmental hazards and toxins, plastics surround me. Until recently, I used my microwave oven daily, often heating things in plastic (big no-no). Finally there is my personal health. I am overweight (BMI of 29) and I love sweets and fatty foods. That is how things stack up on the negative side of the scale.

On the plus side of the scale: I exercise daily, eat loads of vegetables, became vegetarian five years ago and have three grandparents who lived well into their nineties. I meditate, do yoga, relaxation and guided imagery, have an active spiritual life and take time for fun. So why did I get this disease?

Trying to understand why we get this or any other disease, whether there was something we could have done to avoid it, and how to deal with all those feelings of blame, guilt and maybe even shame, is all a normal part of the process. I think everyone who has ever been diagnosed with cancer will bump into the WHY question. The question is: what do you do with it? For me, after struggling with these questions for several days, and realizing that I was getting nowhere, I decided to try to let go of blame, guilt and shame, while holding on to the question of what I could learn from this experience. Clearly, it is not always easy to "just let go," but I do believe that we can make conscious attempts to try to get the better of some of these insidious thoughts and emotions. Making a conscious decision to say "stop" every time I moved in the direction of blame or guilt was helpful. In addition, deciding to focus on listening to the deeper messages of this disease, thinking about what meaning it might have for me, how it could possibly change who I am and who I will become – these were all avenues that I found more worthwhile pursuing. Rather than focus on "why me?", my thoughts became occupied with trying to figure out what to do with this cancer, and how to better live my life on all levels, from the mundane (eat sugar – yes or no?) to the spiritual (daily prayer? meditation?).

A personal note is in order here. I am a believing and practicing Jew. I was raised in a traditional family that ate only kosher food and observed the Sabbath, and I was steeped in Jewish learning and lifestyle from an early age. As I have matured, my Judaism has as well, and while my relationship with God is not always an easy one, the fact that it does exist and it is a relationship I work on, is a central part of who I am today. My struggles with God notwithstanding, during this time of crisis I found that suspending the angst of belief and allowing myself the image of being cradled in God's hand a very comforting thought. I recognize that many of you, my readers, may have difficulty with the notion of a personal God, but if you substitute the words "Higher Power" or "Being" or whatever expression you choose when I write the word God, I think we will understand each other just fine. For those of you who have trouble with that as well, I invite you to skip over the parts that you don't relate to.

But I am getting way ahead of myself. Let's back up to that very first day of living with cancer. In the first hours after diagnosis I felt an adrenaline rush that stayed with me for a couple of hours. I felt as if I had boarded a speed train that was hurtling forward but I did not know the destination. As I drove to Jerusalem and my life flashed by, I fast-forwarded to a deathbed scene, to a funeral. The whole works. I didn't give myself any leeway. I cried along with all the mourners who had come to pay their last respects, but mostly I cried with my children, and for my children who would be motherless. After wallowing in these tears for several long minutes, my natural optimism took over and I mumbled a quiet prayer that I might continue to enjoy my life and family for many years to come.

Arriving in Jerusalem, I met my youngest daughter and gave her a hug that was just a bit stronger and longer than usual. It was clear to me from the outset that while I would tell everybody, and soon, I needed a little time to digest things by myself, and to talk things over with my husband. Yet, how was I to continue acting as if everything was normal when my whole world had just caved in on me? Could I really manage to pull it off and not tell my daughter anything just yet? It turns out that I am a better actress than I ever had imagined. I sailed through the afternoon without arousing any suspicion.

But not telling was extremely stressful for me. My daughter and I went to a coffee shop for a late lunch, and I promptly proceeded to fall apart in a very quiet way. A huge wave of fatigue washed over me and pulled me under. I had never been so tired in my entire life. All I could do was yawn, and keep saying how tired I was. The initial adrenaline rush had worn off and I just wanted to get home and crawl into bed, so I cancelled my next meeting, excusing myself by saying I wasn't feeling well and thankfully my daughter drove us safely home.

Several hours later, with supper dishes put away, and the two teens still living at home busy with their own pursuits, my husband and I grabbed a few precious moments sitting together on the sofa, quietly holding hands. My husband of thirty six years looked at me in a way that he had never looked at me before, as if he was appreciating anew what he might lose. This confirmed for me just how serious this diagnosis was, and how life-threatening. When I caught him looking at me that way over the next couple of weeks I began to joke about it, telling him that he had that "she's dying" look in his eyes, hoping that somehow talking about death and dying might actually chase the fates and demons away. Lucky for me, my husband, the physician, was almost always willing to talk with me about the cancer, and answer the many questions I had. But more on that later.

In contrast to the very sharp and clear recollections from the first few hours after learning about my cancer, my memories of the rest of that day and the next couple of days are a blur. All of a sudden, I entered the medical tunnel of cancer.   Doctor appointments, blood tests, diagnostic tests and more appointments all warped together in slow motion.   Up until then I had been a person who got annual checkups.   Nothing had prepared me for this new stage in life.   My life was tilting crazily, and I was losing my footing.

TIPS FOR THE DAYS FOLLOWING DIAGNOSIS

1. Take time for yourself. Breathe. Walk. Breathe some more.

2. Start a journal and write what is happening to you, what you are thinking and feeling.

3. Speak with someone close to you and with whom you feel comfortable. Share some of your feelings with this friend or family member. You don't have to talk to everybody, or share everything, but choose one or two people with whom you can share openly.

4. Keep to some semblance of your daily routine of meals, sleep time, work and other activities. There is nothing like routine to give us a sense of security and safety. This will help you regain your footing, and give you a sense of life as you know it.

5. Explore using guided imagery to recapture a semblance of safety. For more information on the uses of guided imagery, turn to Chapter 13 right away.

[2]

Sharing the News

Update # 1 – June 24

Hi to my worried family and friends,

I know you are all concerned- and it is tiring to go through this each time- so to simplify for me- I will write an e-mail update and we will go from there. We are figuring our way in this new reality- and I will give this route a try. That is not to say that you can't call, and we can't talk about what is happening, you certainly can, but I think writing group e-mails will make things simpler for me, at least for right now.

After spending the next couple of days adjusting to my new status in life, it was clear to me that the next step was sharing the news – first with my family and then with my co-workers and friends. From the outset, I felt that I had nothing to hide and that I would share everything as fully as possible with both family and friends. This was not a struggle; this came easy to me. Honesty and straightforwardness have been touchstones in my life ever since the time I was five years old and I stole gum from the grocery store.

On that day, when I furtively grabbed a package of gum, something my mother would never agree to buy for me, I felt both shame and guilt. When my mother easily discovered my transgression (I was chewing gum – where did that come from?) she made me march back to the store and hand over the money for the gum. The lesson learned that day, that lying does not pay and honesty is the best policy, have accompanied me through my fifty-six years, and served me well.

I could not imagine the web of lies and subterfuge that would be necessary if I were to try to keep this important news limited to a very small circle of family or friends. Actually, it never occurred to me not to share the news and I have lived comfortably with this decision since Day One.

Having said that, I recognize that this is only one course of action and many folks with cancer choose other ways of dealing with this. Certainly there are considerations with very young children and very old parents that might make this "tell all" policy untenable. Over the course of my cancer journey I have met many wonderful people and, in particular, fellow sojourners on the breast cancer path and I have seen many styles of coping, and the many and varied ways people choose to live their lives with cancer. I would never ever say that you should do exactly what I did, or that there is only one right way. Clearly, that is not so. I did what was right for me, in my particular family constellation, and my personality. When I consider the lessons that I have learned from cancer, probably the most prominent one that has been drilled into my head, repeatedly, is that

"people are different." Now I know that that sounds trivial at best, but no matter how much we all know this to be true, I have somehow come out on the other side of the cancer tunnel with a very deep, almost physical understanding, of just how true this is. So that while for me sharing my news came as naturally as walking or eating, I know that for others this is not the case.

Recently I met a woman who chose to keep the news secret from her parents and sisters. Another woman I met at the day treatment center shared with me that she had not told any of her colleagues at work and thus showed up for work every single day, except for the day she received her chemo, once every other week. Some who do this fear for their job security, others don't want to be pitied, and yet others are embarrassed or feel ashamed. I would argue differently but do not stand in judgment. I merely say that for me this was a very fundamental decision that shaped my entire cancer experience.

On the home front, while it was clear to me that I would share the news about my cancer with my family first, things became quite complicated for a short while when I realized that in three days we would be sending our youngest son, the fifteen-year-old, overseas to a month-long summer camp. The question was: should we tell him before he left for camp? And if we didn't, then when would we tell him? And how? This was a difficult struggle for me. As I said, I hate subterfuge, but didn't want to send him abroad burdened with worry. Thousands of miles would separate us and he might feel very alone and scared. I decided to talk it out with a dear friend of mine, a psychologist, who was once, in his distant past, a camp director. He strongly recommended that we not tell our son before he set out for camp because, to his mind, there were more unknowns than knowns at this point in time, and we were still in the dark as to what my course of treatment would be.

This made some sense to me, and my husband readily agreed. Having decided not to tell my youngest put the whole disclosure bit on hold and my husband and I spent the next three days pretending that in fact our worlds had not fallen apart and it was life as usual. Life as usual at that particular point in time meant that we were due to set out on a month-long vacation in five days' time. Thus, everybody around us was filled with anticipation and questions about our upcoming vacation. Imagine playing the part of excited traveler when inside we knew this trip would never happen, at least not for now. We played along gallantly, all the while thinking that instead of traveling to far-flung locations on the dream vacation we had long planned, the only places we were going to was the doctor's office or hospital. Some vacation indeed.

The weekend before my son left for camp, most of our family assembled to wish both him and us a fond farewell. That had to be the longest weekend in history as far as I was concerned. My husband and I kept up the act and gamely talked about our planned trip, with me taking short breaks to run into the bathroom for a cry. Would anyone notice my red eyes? Apparently not. In fact, although inside I was in turmoil, I discovered yet again that I was a decent actress. Nobody suspected a thing. We got through the weekend and last-minute packing for my son's month at camp without divulging a word about the cancer. After safely depositing him at the airport terminal Sunday morning, I heaved a huge sigh of relief. Now I could focus on how I would share the news with the rest of my children and our parents. Now I could stop pretending and get on with my life.

As I tried to figure out how to tell my children and in what order, I initially pictured myself gathering them all (except the youngest, now off at camp) and sharing the news with all of them at once. I soon realized that it was going to be much too complicated to do it that way, and probably far too dramatic, so I decided to break the news to them one by one. Being the mother of seven children meant that I had seven children to tell, six immediately and one in a month's time. Whom to tell first? How to start? There were so many questions running around my frazzled brain.

I jumped into the water when my second daughter called me that morning to invite me to lunch the next afternoon. My kids know I love to take them out to lunch, and if any one of them has some free time, they give me a call, and if I can get away from my desk I will. I find that these spontaneous lunches are a wonderful time to catch up with each other and they allow for conversations that do not usually happen at larger family gatherings.

We set to meet at Gabriela's, my favorite Italian restaurant, located on a pedestrian mall in downtown Jerusalem. The setting is picturesque, with old stone buildings framing the walkway, and the Italian food is wonderful. Only this time I doubted that I would have much of an appetite. As we sat down, and before we could even have a look at the menu, I could not hold back and blurted out my news without any preamble or warning. "I have some bad news to share with you. I have breast cancer." After my daughter's look of shock passed, and we ordered stuffed mushrooms and salmon, we spent the rest of lunch talking about IT and I answered all the questions she could think of as best I could, withholding nothing. I asked her to let me talk to her sibs one by one and give them the news myself before she talked with them. I knew this would be hard for her, and actually the trickiest part of telling the kids one by one. They were their own natural support system and, since I could not tell them all at once, I needed them to wait a few days before I could complete my rounds and that support could kick in.

Many people have asked me how my children reacted. That question has both puzzled me and made me feel uncomfortable because I did not know how to answer it. Looking back, I think I was   so involved in my own situation that it was hard for me to gauge just how my children reacted and how they were coping with the knowledge that their mom had cancer. They seemed to be doing okay, but I didn't really know nor did I stop to check. The tables were turned. Rather than being "mother hen" worrying about how my kids were doing, it was time for them to monitor how I was doing, and to mother me. I was so overwhelmed with my new state of affairs that I had few reserves left for anybody else. It was my time to focus on me. They would be fine.

Looking back with the perspective of time, what is my memory of my children's immediate responses to my news? Not surprisingly, each one reacted differently. One cried, one was quiet, most asked a lot of questions. Even though emotionally I was less available to them, and more focused on myself, I was secure in the knowledge that they had each other to talk to and to   offer   support   one   to   the other, which is certainly an advantage of having a large, cohesive family. I told each one of my children that they could ask   me anything at all and that I would try to tell them everything and hold nothing back. I knew that I was building on long-established, strong relationships of open and honest communication. They have all let me know in one way or another that setting the tone of honesty and openness made it much easier for them.

I traveled far and wide to share the news with my children over the next couple of days, and although my efforts were sincere, mistakes were made.   My biggest mistake, in perfect hindsight, was telling one of my sons over the phone. Why did I choose to tell him by phone when clearly face-to-face was the method of choice?   By week's end, five of the kids had been told   the   news,   and   the   only remaining son in the country was in the far north of Israel, working as a youth counselor with a group of visiting Australian youth. He was not scheduled for time off at home for another week.   My dilemma was whether to tell him by phone or to wait an entire week and tell him in person. I decided to break the news by phone, thinking that the chances that he might hear from someone other than me were too great. Mistake. Big mistake. I was looking after my own needs rather than his. I wanted to finish the arduous task of breaking the news. I also did not want him to feel left out. What I did not take into account was that he was in a responsible position, far from home, without a support network of his own to help him out. He received the news like a cold shower, and immediately had to go back to work without a minute to catch his breath. Later he told me how difficult this had been for him, to be all alone with no one to talk to.

He felt isolated from the family and confused but at the same time, responsible to his very demanding job. He is a strong young man (both emotionally and physically) and he dealt with it okay. However, in retrospect, if I had to do it again, I   would   make   the major effort to travel the three hours in each direction to share the news with him in person or else wait a week, and ask everybody else to keep it quiet.

And what about my youngest son in summer camp overseas? We kept the news from him as long as we could. I was in direct communication with the camp and the directors knew exactly what was going on with me over the course of the month. Together, we decided to hold off sharing the news with my son as long as possible. At the end of almost four weeks, before going into surgery, I felt strongly that it was time to break the news to him. After consulting once again with the camp directors, I called my son and over the crackling phone line, with him sounding like he was at the other end of the world, I gave him only the barest details over phone. I told him that I had had some medical tests and that I had to have some minor surgery. I had decided not to even mention the "C word." Wouldn't you know it? The first question he asked me was, "Is it cancer?" I, of course, answered truthfully. He later told me that upon hearing the news he was in shock for a few hours, feeling totally "out of it", but after a short time he was able to get back to the business of being a camper as usual. As it was, he was at the beginning of a rocky time in adolescence and throwing him this curve ball was not the nicest or smartest thing to do but, then again, I hadn't asked for this cancer either.

You might wonder why telling my children in person was so important to me. Why did I make the efforts I did, and why did I struggle so much with the two sons that I could not tell in person? Primarily, I think, so that my kids could see that I was really okay. I looked the same as I had the week before. I felt fine. I did not feel sick. By looking into their eyes and being there with them, I was able to reassure them as best as I could and promise that I would share with them all the information I had. Seeing that Mom looked and acted more or less the same had to be reassuring at such a scary time. Cancer is such a grim diagnosis with so many dim possibilities. At the outset, a diagnosis of cancer associates directly with DEATH. I can imagine that my children were beginning to conjure up life without Mom, and my painful and slow demise. In fact, cancer in this day and age is often more like a chronic disease that one learns to live with. This was something that we would all learn about in the future. Right now, we were dealing with that life-threatening, terribly scary diagnosis: Cancer.

Now that my family knew as much as I did, I began to move on to friends and colleagues. How much to share and with whom are very pertinent questions. When you enter the cancer world,   as   you undergo your trial by fire, there is a lot of information flying around, a lot of hypotheses, maybes, what ifs and unknowns. Who needs to know what? How much detail is the right amount?

My policy was to share with my family and friends the facts that we had at the moment. I did not share with them all the potentials, the possibilities, and the doomsday scenarios. That I did with my husband, Mike, and believe me, I analyzed these thoroughly with him. By that I mean that I regularly reviewed with him all the things that could go wrong, often revisiting grim fates, statistics notwithstanding. Even though the odds were strongly in my favor, it felt to me that discussing all possibilities, even the grimmer ones, with Mike somehow calmed me down. For me it was important to have one person I could lay everything out with. My good luck was that my life's companion is a knowledgeable physician, a caring human being and a best friend. With him, I hashed and rehashed all of the less-than-pleasant possibilities. With my immediate family, I shared the current facts, and the expected next step or two. As more knowledge became available, and a treatment plan took shape, I was able to share with them what was happening and what the immediate plan was.

I realized one day, about two weeks after my diagnosis that one could actually go overboard in terms of sharing and openness. My awareness came about after bumping into an old acquaintance in the supermarket. This was somebody I had a friendly but superficial relationship with, and I had not seen her in a long time. She asked me in the way that people do when they have not seen each other in a while "How are you?" That was all of an opening that I needed. I immediately told her that I had been diagnosed with breast cancer. When I saw her face fall, I realized that this sharing might be taking things a bit too far. Perhaps I did not have to share this piece of news with everybody at all times. I tried to tone things down a bit after that, and to be a bit more judicious about the casual "how are you's?" in the supermarket aisles. Nevertheless, I felt a strong need to share my news far and wide with friends, neighbors, colleagues and extended family, and so I did.

For those who wonder, "Why share at all?" I believe that there are several good reasons to be open about this kind of news. The first has to do with support. Of all of the qualities and characteristics that help build resilience, social support has been shown to be the strongest, most significant factor in study after study. So, clearly, social support is a good thing.

The net result of my sharing the news with friends and family was that I was overwhelmed with an outpouring of care of every imaginable kind, from love to physical help and back to emotional support. The waves of love I felt from family and friends were both heartwarming and amazingly wonderful. These included offers of rides, deliveries of hot soup, muffins, and casseroles to my doorstep and, most important of all, the visits, all of which nourished my body and soul.

Since my children are grown and housekeeping chores are at a minimum, I needed less physical support than many other people who are diagnosed with cancer. People who have cancer often have physical needs that may include child care, housecleaning, dealing with bureaucracy, and actual physical care. I was fortunate to have a weekly house cleaner and a very able husband who picked up a lot of the household slack, allowing me to take care of myself without feeling burdened by household chores. Physical and emotional supports were both helpful and heartwarming, but what surprised me most was the feeling I got from knowing that people were praying for me. Growing up in a religious tradition and believing in the power of prayer, I have been intrigued by the recent psychological and medical journals that have studied intercessory prayer and have come up with some tantalizing results. By sharing my news with my many circles of acquaintance from family to colleagues to friends, many of whom asked if they could pray for me, I found that I was indeed strengthened by the knowledge that people in far-flung corners of the world were praying for my recovery. At one point I joked that God must be wondering, "Who is this Naomi Chava daughter of Chaya Hendel that I am hearing so much about?" (In the Jewish tradition, the supplicant's prayers for healing are phrased as the sick person's name with the appendage of their mother's name).

My feelings about being the object of prayer actually evolved over the course of the year. In the beginning of my cancer journey, when someone would tell me that they were praying for me it would catch me off guard and I often felt a flicker of embarrassment. Up until now, this was something I did for other people. Now people were doing this for me. Over the period of a few months, I learned to turn that feeling around and soak it up, feeling blessed from the very notion that people were praying for me and sending me good wishes. Just yesterday, when I called to schedule my annual mammography appointment (the momentous first one AFTER treatment), the secretary told me that she thinks of me every day – a code word for telling me that she prays for me daily. Over the year, I met many people who told me I was in their prayers. What a wonderful feeling it was for me to feel surrounded, protected and supported by people who love me and were sending their prayers heavenward.

As part of my effort to be open and to share with family and friends, I began to write e-mail updates. Initially the list of recipients was just my immediate family, and the reason I wrote to them was to make sure that they all knew what was happening and that I had not left anyone out. In our large family, it has happened on more than one occasion that somebody missed some important news. I did not want this to happen now, yet I found that I was getting tired of repeating the same thing over and over again. While I appreciated everyone's concern and interest, and really did want to share what was going on with me, I did not want to spend all day on the phone. Over time, in addition to physical reports about what was going on medically speaking, the e-mails became a way to share with family and friends my thoughts, feelings and experiences, as well as another way to receive a tremendous outpouring of support. For every e-mail I sent, I got many, many heartwarming ones in return. I share many of my e-mail missives in this book (usually at the beginning of a chapter) so that you can appreciate in "real time" what I was going through, what I was thinking and how I was feeling. While this book is retrospective, those e-mails were written in the trenches as I was experiencing the day-to-day trials of cancer.

TIPS ON SHARING THE NEWS

1. Do it in person.

2. Keep the details short and pertinent.

3. Decide with whom you want to share the news with and how much you want to share. This is up to you. This may also change over time.

4. If somebody asks you about something that you do not wish to divulge, tell them in a straightforward manner that you would rather not talk about it. Remember: you get to decide whom you tell and how much.

[3]

Finding Your Footing

Update # 2 - June 30

Another two weeks probably of being in this in-between state. We are doing well all things considered. Mike and I continue to exercise, work, and go out – we have a wedding of a neighbor to attend next week, and will undoubtedly see a movie or two. If possible we may take a couple of days to go scuba diving down south (we are trying to keep Wed-Fri clear, but if the MRI comes along we will grab it) – so we are taking more or less each day as it comes.

I am happy for "dates", entertainment, creative suggestions for joint activities :)) as well as friendly letters and calls. I can't always answer your calls right away but text messages are great too.

I know that your thoughts and prayers are with me and it means the world.

I am going about my days in what i call emergency routine   i.e. going to work, the grocery store, etc. It sounds like daily routine, but now it is all done against the backdrop of the big "C".   Of course there are many interruptions for tests and appointments – all related to my new "career" – it really does feel like a substantial full time job I have taken upon myself.

As the days wore on and things were still very much up in the air regarding how to treat my cancer, my days began to have a new shape and outline. My waking hours were filled with phone calls, scheduling, paperwork, tests, and here and there a little bit of work thrown in for good measure. I tried to continue some semblance of my regular routine, recognizing as a truth what I knew from my professional life, that in times of crisis, routine gives us a sense of security and comfort. It was not always easy, but doing the things that I always did – exercise, grocery shopping and cooking dinners - made me feel "normal", during this time when my whole world had turned upside down and nothing else seemed normal at all.

Initially, I thought it would be so simple. I had breast cancer. They would cut out what needed to be cut out, and we would go from there. Was I ever wrong. First, we had to find out where the cancer was located. Because my diagnosis was made on the basis of a lymph node biopsy, and I had no discernible breast mass, we embarked on a hunt-and-destroy mission to find the primary site of the cancer. My days were filled with scheduling tests and then waiting patiently, or impatiently, until the appointed hour arrived. Additional mammograms came up negative, which led to a breast MRI, and subsequent to that an MRI biopsy, which means a biopsy done while undergoing an additional MRI. All of this was in addition to a host of other diagnostic and imaging tests to rule out metastases in various other body parts.

When I got back my first set of blood tests after the initial diagnosis was made, I wasn't quite sure where to put them so that I would be able to find them if needed. When had I ever needed   to   save medical records before? I quickly realized that this situation was different and organization would be key. Making the appointments, getting the insurance paperwork done, and the HMO bureaucracies sorted out was almost a full-time job and required high-level organizational skills as well.

I decided to this end that an accordion folder with ten or more sections to hold various medical reports, insurance forms, referrals, lab work, test results and anything else that might crop up was just the thing I needed. I hopped over to the local stationery store to make the purchase, and the helpful clerk offered me a black folder. A BLACK folder! Gulp! Deathly black. Catching me totally by surprise, tears immediately rose to the surface and I almost broke down right then and there. Mustering what little self-control I had left, in a shaky voice I asked the clerk if she had the folders in stock in any other color, and held my breath. Luckily for me, she rummaged around and found a bright blue one. It seems so trivial, but I just could not stomach the idea of using a black folder; it seemed somehow to augur doom. I needed to use all of my reserves to convince myself that I would come out of this tunnel one day on the other side, and be okay.

It is surprising how often the little things that you least expect to, set you off, while the seemingly much greater challenges are sailed through. It may be that the greater challenges are more readily
apparent, and can be mentally prepared for. Rehearsing how I will behave in a certain situation or what I might say can help

me get ready for the challenge. It is those little, unexpected things that you can't prepare for, and often knock you for a loop.

As the days progressed, I clocked a lot of hospital time going for   a variety of diagnostic tests and procedures. Of all of the tests that I did, the first breast MRI was the most upsetting. In trying to understand why, I believe it had to do with the medical personnel and the way they treated me. Now I realize that most of you are not in the field of medicine but I feel that this is worth relating, in the hopes that you can learn from my experience and become more assertive, stick up for yourselves, and thus be spared some of the indignities I experienced.

So here's the scene: after being directed to change into a hospital gown, and having an IV catheter placed in my arm, the female MRI tech asked me to lie face down on the gurney in front of the MRI machine, making sure that each one of my breasts fitted into the metal forms on the gurney. Without explaining what she was doing or why, she then tied my arms behind me with masking tape. She did not ask me if I was comfortable. She did not reassure me. She told me under no uncertain terms that I was not to move and that the test would take at least twenty minutes. I felt as if I was in a straitjacket. I kept flashing to images of "One Flew over the Cuckoo's Nest" with Nurse Ratched in attendance. I timidly asked   if   I   could   listen   to music with earphones during the procedure, and was curtly told, "No." The stretcher that I was lying on began to move slowly into the MRI machine, which made a terrific noise and was very hot. Apparently, the ventilation wasn't working that day, or the technician didn't feel that it was necessary to put the fan on. I felt like I was inside a washing machine, and my head was going round and round. I had the sense that the machine was closed at one end (it wasn't, but I couldn't see that), increasing my claustrophobic tendencies. I began to feel extremely anxious. I tried breathing. I tried guided imagery. My muscles were cramping up. How many more minutes to go? Why weren't they telling me?

Finally, Nurse Ratched said, "Seven minutes to go." Only thirteen minutes had passed? How could that be? It seemed like an eternity, an hour at the very least. My brain was screaming let me out of here. I tried breathing again, slowly in, and even more slowly out. "Focus on the breathing," I told myself. "Use all the skills you have." That worked for about ten seconds. Finally the MRI was finished. I was extricated from the machine, and from the straitjacket. When I exclaimed how unpleasant the experience had been, Nurse Ratched let me know, again in no uncertain terms, how grateful I should be. "Getting an MRI is not something to be taken for granted," she said. Thanks a lot for the lesson on gratitude.

After that experience, my upcoming second MRI, which was to take forty minutes because of the biopsy they were planning to do during the MRI, loomed threateningly on the horizon. If the twenty-minute MRI was excruciating, how would I last through forty minutes? What could I do to prepare myself? I could not think of a thing. I obsessed.

Fortunately, it was an entirely different experience. I came expecting the worst, and instead was pleasantly surprised. The attending physician, a bright young woman, explained everything to me thoroughly, helped me feel that I was partner to the process, and touched my back several times during the MRI, inquiring in a very caring fashion how I was doing. Moreover, this time the ventilation was much better and, before beginning the procedure, I carefully looked at the MRI machine noting that it was open at both ends, so I didn't feel quite so claustrophobic. My hands were not tied nor taped down so the feeling of being an incarcerated psychiatric patient was gone. The forty minutes passed much more quickly than I had anticipated, the staff was pleasant and encouraging, and this time when I got off the gurney, I was indeed grateful.

From these two very different MRIs, I learned the following – most of which should be obvious, but is worth re-stating.

Things I would like to tell the medical staff:

1. Talk to your patients. Explain to them what is happening and what they can expect.

2. Treat your patients like human beings.

3. Don't be afraid to touch your patient on the arm or back. Research shows how healing touch can be.

And to you, dear reader, don't be afraid to ask the medical staff what to expect and how long it will take. Additionally, if you are feeling discomfort or pain, speak up!

Update # 3 - July 7

The most significant event since my last update is the MRI
biopsy I did yesterday, completing all the tests that I need to do, at least for now. I was originally supposed to do the test on Sunday, but got a call that the machine was broken. After my initial disappointment, I realized that it could always be worse....I could have been IN the machine with a needle stuck inside of me when it broke down. You have to be thankful for the little (and big) things and I am.

So now we are waiting, and while this period of uncertainty is certainly stretching out longer than I might have thought, I find that it has given me some time to catch my breath, to appreciate all the wonderful things and people (I should say people and things) I have in my life, and to continue enjoying them, minute by minute, day by day.

Assembling Your Team

When I was first diagnosed with breast cancer, I pictured myself as "IT" in the children's game where you are blindfolded and spun around and around so that you lose any sense of where you are. The spinning leaves you off balance, and without landmarks to guide you as you stumble around trying to make your way. That is how I felt. But as the days passed, I slowly began to regain my balance. A crucial piece in regaining my balance was assembling a medical team. In addition to my family physician, I now needed a surgeon and an oncologist. I had so many questions: Did they have to be at the same hospital or on the same team? When was I to visit them? Would they talk to each other? Were second opinions in order? How was I to find answers to all these and many more questions?

For different people there will be different answers. This is the time to tap into the medical resources you do have. Friends and family members can be helpful; internet may be of some use. However, for most of us, our family physician or GP is the one we will turn to for guidance. My family physician stepped up to the plate, as well as my physician husband, and both were able to guide me through the maze. For many, a patient advocate may be the answer. It is clear to me that keeping your wits about you, staying focused and more organized than you have ever been in your life, and building a treatment plan - all while your world is crumbling around you - is an almost impossible task.   Recruiting friends and family members to help at this critical time can be very helpful to you. Don't forget that it will be helpful to them as well, as all of us feel so helpless in the face of cancer and this allows those closest to us to DO something.

As I began to narrow in on a surgeon and oncologist, I decided that I wanted to meet and talk with both of them very early in the game, before much of the data from the tests I was doing was in. Even though I was told that there was time, I was eager to get this show on the road and needed to know who would be taking care of me. I preemptively made appointments with doctors who had come highly recommended, not waiting to be told that it was time to see them. I wanted to make sure that the recommended doctors were in fact the right ones for me, and I wanted to move quickly once the data was in. I have never been a patient person.

What was important to me in choosing a physician? First and foremost was that the doctor should have an excellent reputation, experience, and a broad knowledge base.   In addition, the things that were important to me were availability, openness, willingness to talk and listen, and accessibility. In choosing my doctors, I needed to determine whether I had confidence in them, could talk to them, and be assured of being heard and getting the answers I needed. I cannot underscore enough how important I think this is. I believe that trust and confidence form the cornerstone of the healing alliance between doctor and patient, and if I feel good with my physicians and have confidence in them, the healing process can proceed.

I came armed with many questions about my disease and treatment options, but also asked about accessibility and how the decision-making process was handled. I felt that I was actually interviewing my physicians before letting them on to my team. Both the oncologist and the surgeon gave me their cell phone numbers and their e-mails. I was surprised by how open they were and how easy the access would be. While I called no more than once or twice during the entire year, the knowledge that my physicians were just a phone call away was highly reassuring. Once I had met the physicians and found them both to my liking, I felt another ring of support growing around me and calming me down.

In addition to choosing individual physicians whom I liked and had confidence in, it was important to me for the surgeon and oncologist to communicate with each other directly. That would seem obvious, but unfortunately, it is not something to be taken for granted. It is important to ascertain how the various physicians on your team will communicate, and whether they know and respect each other. I ended up choosing a medical facility that had weekly interdisciplinary meetings with the oncologist, breast surgeon and radiologist, all present, along with the breast cancer nurse. This assured me that, while there might be differences of opinion among the various members of the team, we were all listening to each other and taking into consideration the same things.

The breast cancer nurse was the one person I did not choose. She came along with the surgeon and oncologist and was a blessing from heaven. Susan, the nurse at the hospital where I was treated, was knowledgeable, reassuring and very accessible. From the moment I met her she helped me, in her very no-nonsense way, navigate the system and figure out what I had to do next. Her job description, as far as I can tell, is to help smooth the road of the breast cancer patient and make sure that nobody gets lost in the shuffle. In many ways she functioned more like a social worker, but with the added value of having extensive medical knowledge about breast cancer.

As I entered the medical world of breast cancer, what I began to realize was that medicine is more of an art form than a science. As the wife of a doctor for well over 35 years, this was an idea that was not entirely new to me. However, the reality of this struck home particularly hard now, as we were trying to figure out what I had and how to treat IT, whatever IT was. One might have thought that a diagnosis of cancer brings with it a clear course of treatment. Often things are not quite so well defined, and being able to sift through the data, the research and the treatment options all at the same time is where science and art merge.

TIPS ON CREATING YOUR TREATMENT PLAN

1. Be proactive. Seek out information about your disease, find excellent health providers in your area and locate medical centers that have experience in dealing with your disease.

2. Become organized. Even if this doesn't come naturally to you, you will be dealing with lots of paperwork, forms, test results, etc. Buy a   big accordion folder (not black!) with several sections. Put all test results, letters and consultation notes in it. Save everything.

3. If you are not good at organization, or are simply feeling overwhelmed, get a friend or family member to help you with paperwork, appointment scheduling, and anything else you might need. I have found that in general, people want to help, and if given a specific job, are often grateful.

4. Ask all the questions of your doctor that you want. Do not be afraid, ashamed or embarrassed. He or she is there for you, and that is their job.

5. Make sure you feel comfortable with the doctors you have chosen. If you are not comfortable, consider changing. You are the client. You should be satisfied.

6. Bring someone with you to all doctor appointments. It is very good to have two sets of ears hearing everything that the doctor is

saying. **Often it may be hard for you, the patient,   to** actually hear the details of what the doctor is saying. Bringing along someone who can take notes about the meeting can be most helpful later when reviewing what has happened, and what will happen next.

7. Consider hiring a patient advocate. In some countries there are non-profit volunteer organizations that provide these patient advocates. In other areas you can hire someone to help you manage your case. Either way, your "Cancer Guide" should be able to help you navigate the system, whether it is scheduling appointments, talking to doctors, or getting social security benefits.

[4]

Surgery

Update #4 - July 18

Got the biopsy results that showed that in fact I do have ductal cell carcinoma - in situ. This may or may not explain the lymph node. So.... Today I went and did an experimental imaging test, called MBI (you can read up on it on the web if you are so inclined), there will be some results tomorrow. Tomorrow I also have an appointment with the surgeon to discuss "things" and maybe figure out next steps. Many of you have asked how I am holding out- whether I am feeling impatient, etc. I am surprisingly patient- surprising, because I am not a very patient person in general. So why am I patient now- two hypotheses: 1. All the guided imagery and meditation is kicking in and changing my personality or....2. None of the prospects are too exciting: surgery-chemo-radiation.

I still don't know which of the above it will be- how long, how much, etc etc- all remain a big question mark.

After close to a month of tests and waiting for lab results, the results were finally in. A small mass had been located in my right breast that seemed to be the original source of the cancer. Maybe. In any case, my team was assembled and now the decision had to be made: what kind of surgery was it to be? A lumpectomy or the dreaded mastectomy? Lumpectomy is a more minor surgery in which the offending cancer is cut out along with a minimal amount of surrounding tissue. In my case the lymph nodes would also be removed, no matter which type of surgery I chose. A mastectomy is a more radical type of surgery in which the entire breast is removed, but even within that category there are the more extensive and less extensive procedures to choose from.

Deciding among surgical options was both difficult and anxiety provoking. The first surgeon I consulted with, whom I liked
immediately, recommended lumpectomy, although he did say mastectomy was an option, should I wish to do that. He performed surgery in a local hospital with a strong oncology department, so the cards were definitely in his favor. Nevertheless, I decided to get a second opinion, since my case wasn't straightforward (is there ever such a thing as a straightforward case?) The second surgeon I consulted, who practiced in a different hospital in another town, agreed that lumpectomy would be her first choice. I breathed a sigh of relief, mixed with worry.

Why worry? Why wasn't this a simple, straightforward decision? They both weighed in on the side of lumpectomy. I should   be
dancing for joy. But I wasn't. Initially the thought of a mastectomy totally blew me away. I tried to picture myself minus a breast. Then I pictured myself minus two breasts. It was scary. It was more than scary. I gingerly entered the world of internet to see what it might look like and hear what people were saying about the decades-long debate of lumpectomy vs.

mastectomy. What I found was: a) too much information b) a lot of inaccurate information and c) nobody who spoke to my very specific situation. But my readings about mastectomy had led me to believe that if I removed my breast, I would be getting rid of all possibility of future breast cancer on the side that was removed. That sounded good. Actually, that sounded great! I thought to myself, "Let's remove both of them. Who needs them?" I was all ready to go for a bilateral mastectomy, so I checked back with my ever-available surgeon for a chat. He informed me that while a bilateral mastectomy would reduce the chance of recurrence by a certain percentage, I could still get cancer on my chest wall. In addition, since I wasn't a BRCA carrier (breast cancer gene) there were no indications for removing both breasts and he, for one, wouldn't do it. So I was back to square one. Lumpectomy or mastectomy? What would it be? The doctors had given me all the information I needed, they had given me their recommendations, but they had also told me very clearly that this was a very personal decision and it was up to me to decide. According to both surgeons, both options were feasible and if I were to choose a mastectomy they would have no difficulties performing it.

So I struggled, and the thoughts went round and round in my feverish brain. While both surgeons had weighed in on the side of lumpectomy I still wasn't convinced. Would I have better chances of survival if I did a mastectomy? Was that the brave thing to do? Would I be sorry five years down the road? How to decide? I struggled back and forth with the issue. If I had the more radical surgery I would reduce chances of recurrence by a very small percentage. Did I need that safety margin? Who could tell me? On the other hand, if I had the mastectomy, how would it affect my quality of life? I tried turning the decision over to Mike and, while he was willing to discuss all the pros and cons ad nauseum, he refused to decide for me.

After sleeping on it, thinking about it, talking and talking and talking about it, I finally made my decision by falling back to default mode. Default mode for me as a rule is the less intervention, the better. Thus, the smaller, less invasive surgery won out, and the die was cast. Lumpectomy it would be.

Surgery was quickly scheduled for five days later and, because I had taken care of pre-op matters earlier in the month, there was little to do but wait. Hurry up and wait. Since Mike and I felt robbed of our well-deserved month-long vacation, we had decided to take advantage of every small stretch of time we had to get away. Earlier in the month we had gone on a two-night getaway to a boutique hotel near Safed in the northern part of Israel. Now we decided to return to one of our favorite haunts, the sulphur springs at Hamat Gader, on the Jordanian/Syrian border, for an overnight.

I found that getting away for short breaks from the new routine of doctor appointments, tests, phone calls and well-meaning friends and family was a breath of fresh air. For a few minutes or hours, I could almost forget that there was something terribly wrong with me. Keep in mind that, thankfully, the cancer wasn't affecting how I felt physically. I still felt the same as I always had. I even looked the same. I was strong, healthy, and had a good appetite. There was no way that anyone would ever think that I was ILL. That I had CANCER! Leaving it all behind for a few days was a very real way to step out of my new identity as a cancer patient, and return to being my old familiar self. It was a blessed relief, and something that

I highly recommend to those of you reading this book who have cancer. Even if you feel that you must keep the home fires burning, try to find a way to take even a few hours off from cancer, whether it is a walk in the woods, a massage, or a movie. Cancer tends to permeate every area of your life, and getting a break feels good, and if it feels good, to my mind, it has got to be healing. Reminding yourself that you had a life before cancer, and hopefully you will have one after cancer, is restorative.

During our day and night at the sulfur springs, I succeeded in keeping thoughts of the future at bay until we began our drive home. Speaking to Susan, the breast cancer nurse, in the car on the way home, I was pulled up short and vacation mode quickly vanished. As we talked about what to expect over the next couple of days, Susan suddenly mentioned the word chemo. CHEMO. It pierced my consciousness. Early on, the surgeon had told me I would definitely need surgery and radiation, and that chemo was a possibility to be determined at a later date. I had immediately pushed all thoughts of chemo underground. For whatever reason, when Susan now mentioned chemo, it dawned upon me that it was a real and present possibility and that thought, along with the impending surgery, sent me into a palpable downward spiral. My good mood evaporated into thin air and I was flooded with thoughts of "what if" and "maybe", the familiar and anxious terrain of cancer patients.

As I write these words, it is hard for me to convey just how surprised I was with the notion of chemo in relation to me. How, you ask, could I possibly have ignored that possibility, and how could it be a surprise? The human ability to live in a state of denial is quite remarkable, and very often it is just that denial that allows us the time we need to prepare ourselves for what is to come. I recently was witness to a woman suffering from pancreatic cancer who successfully avoided talking about what she had for many, many months. She was perfectly happy continuing her life as it had been, taking care of what she absolutely had to, but not dealing with the impending implications of late stage pancreatic cancer. Denial was helping her cope. Denial is what helped me get through those first few weeks after diagnosis. When I was ready to hear about chemo, I was able to slowly begin to acknowledge the more-than-likely possibility that I would be a candidate. That isn't to say I was happy about it. To the contrary. I felt sad, unhappy, and lethargic; all legitimate emotions that people often experience when encountering difficulty. My negative reaction to the possibility of chemo evaporated after several hours, when I was able to once again suppress thoughts of it, until the next time it would rear its ugly head several weeks down the road.

Upon return from our overnight vacation, with just a few days to go, I decided that it was time to prepare myself for the upcoming surgery. Shuffling through piles of papers, I located the explanatory pages about the surgery that I had not looked at since receiving them at the pre-op session at the hospital, and tried to recall what Susan had told me to expect about the surgery. My mind was a blank. If there was anything I was supposed to do or to remember, it was gone. The explanatory pages were moderately helpful, but overall I felt as if I was walking into unknown territory with my eyes closed.

The day of surgery dawned bright and hot. The plan was for me to go first thing in the morning to the mammography clinic to get "marked" so that the surgeon would know exactly what and

how much to remove. I needed to get there before their regular day
 started. I had been warned by both friends and medical staff that this could be a painful procedure. I was then supposed to check in to the hospital. Since my surgery wasn't scheduled until the mid-afternoon I was told not to get there before noon, leaving me at least two hours with nothing to do. What worried me more than the pain of the marking procedure was the two hours to kill with pins sticking out of my breast before checking in for surgery. What was I going to do with all this time?? Normal distractions such as going for breakfast at a coffee shop wouldn't work because I was on a pre-op fast.   A museum?   Out of the question with pins sticking out of my boobs. What was I going to do??

My daughters saved the day for me, assuring me that they would be with me the whole time and we would figure it out as we went. They joined me for my early morning appointment at the
mammography clinic. One of my daughters took the meaning of solidarity to new heights. She insisted that she would go braless if I had to be without my bra so that I wouldn't feel alone. Fortunately we didn't have to test her loyalty. After the marking procedure, which was not nearly as painful as anticipated, two of my sons joined the festivities. They had decided to join in later in the morning, feeling that the mammography clinic was a particularly female venue and one they would not feel comfortable in. So off the five of us went to a small nature reserve, where we hung out and dangled our feet in the water of a natural spring for the two hours we had to kill. We joked, told stories, and easily passed the time I had so dreaded. The solidarity and support I felt from my children on that particular morning was remarkable. It was clear to me that

the need to be with each other was mutual. They needed to be with me almost as much as I needed to be with them, yet their ability to be there for me just when I needed them, and just how I needed them, amazed me. They were there in ways that only they could be and I was immensely grateful.

At noon we made our way to the hospital, where the kids continued to distract me with games they had brought along to make the wait more bearable. We set up a card table in the hallway and proceeded to play "Set" and "Taboo" until it was almost surgery time. Aside from a couple of dirty looks from the nursing staff after a particularly rowdy round, the time passed. At the appointed hour Mike arrived, the nurse led me to my bed and I was given a valium, which I happily downed. I then proceeded to listen to my guided imagery scripts for surgery on my MP3 player (more on that in Chapter 13), which kept me calm as I was prepped and then wheeled off to the operating room.

Waking up from surgery a few hours later, I found myself with a large bandage over my right breast and a drain for fluids coming out of my side. I didn't feel much pain. Fortunately, the general anesthetic cleared my system easily and I felt well almost immediately, so much so that I was quite hungry just a couple of hours after surgery. I know that many folks suffer nausea or worse, but I was lucky and seemed to sail through that piece. Lucky for me there was a sushi bar right around the corner from the hospital and my daughter happily delivered take-out dinner for all of us. Sushi sure beats hospital food.

Early the next morning I was up and writing at my computer. I sent out the following letter from my hospital bed:

Update #6 - July 25

Hi all- Just a quick note to let you know that I had surgery yesterday afternoon. All went well, as far as I know. I have not seen the surgeon yet although Mike saw him yesterday after surgery. I feel pretty good– I am walking and talking. Since Mike is a strong proponent of pain relief when necessary, he encouraged me to take pain pills, which I did. Personally, I prefer beer and wine but as far as I know they don't do that IV. Now I heal and wait, or as my good friend Janis says "hurry up and wait" which characterizes quite well this new stage of life. Now we wait for the path results to come back before we figure out the next steps.

I ended up going home midday, less than 24 hours after surgery, at my husband's urgings. He was worried about infection, since the roommates on either side of me both had serious infections. The bright midday sun burned down on us on the drive home, and I immediately started dreaming of air conditioning. I knew that I would be spending a fair amount of time up in my bedroom and decided then and there that after 19 years of living in our house without AC, now was the time to install air conditioning in our bedroom. In the car on the way home, I called and placed the order. The air rconditioner was on the way and I was feeling cooler already.

I realize that my modus operandi is action. I like to be in control, I like to move and do. It is hard to catch me in a restful moment of repose. That may be quite different than the way you approach the world and your cancer. This is a good time to reiterate that everybody is different and what works for one, doesn't work for all.

The recuperation period from surgery was fairly uneventful except for the drain. Nobody had actually mentioned to me that there would be a drain and, since I had never had surgery before, it wasn't something that I was even aware of. I realize that a drain does not seem like a big deal to a surgeon, or to surgical nurses. Just about everybody who has surgery gets a drain. They abound on surgical floors. However, to a patient a drain is a pain in more ways than one. How do you go anywhere with this bottle that keeps filling up with red tinged fluid? How do you hide it? And the nagging worry about when is it ever going to stop draining? It seemed to me that mine was filling up more and more as the time went by, and smelling worse and worse. Over the next three weeks I chose clothes that had pockets so that I could hide the bottle in a pocket with long tunics covering the hose. Most people were not aware that I even had the drain, but it was a constant, nagging thought in my mind. Cleaning out the collection bottle was a daily chore that I found harder and harder to bear as the time went on. I worried about the smell. I worried that I would be attached to this thing forever. It pulled at my skin and was uncomfortable when I lay down, adding to my difficulties with sleeping. While sex was not at the top of my list of favorite activities after surgery, being constantly aware of the state of my drain did not add to my waning libido. Learning to live with the drain did not become easier with time, although I think that only I was affected by it; it didn't really bother anybody around me. By the three week mark I had had it and, although I was still leaking, I think the surgeon had had it too, and he pulled the damn thing out.

Update #7-July 28

> *As for my recuperation: I feel pretty good – a little beat up, a little tired, sometimes cranky by the end of the day. But all in all I think I am doing alright. Visits, flowers, muffins, letters, and get well cards have all arrived in exactly the right amounts, letting me know that people care about me and love me, and that feels very very good.*

Now, more than a year later, when I think back to the surgery, about the only thing that I remember clearly is the drain and how much I hated it. When the surgeon finally pulled it out, he warned me that I might leak a little bit out of the hole where the drain had been attached. Did he say "a little"?? I felt like I was having a period from my drain hole for at least two weeks after it was removed. Every morning I packed the side of my bra with gauze pads, as advised by the doctor, and when they leaked through after just a short time, I switched to actual sanitary napkins. It really was a period! I could not imagine how it was ever going to stop leaking and dry up. But one day it finally did.

Once the drain was pulled and the hole finally stopped leaking, I started obsessing about lymphedema. During my surgery, in addition to the lumpectomy, I had twenty-two lymph nodes removed. One of the side effects I was warned about was lymphedema. Lymphedema, put simply, is swelling of tissue cause by some kind of blockage in the lymph transport system. You may not know this (I certainly did not before this point in time) but parallel to the circulatory system of the blood, you and I have a lymph circulatory system where there are approximately three liters of lymph circulating at any given time.

Much of what had been draining out of my hole had been lymphatic fluid. I figured that all that fluid that had been draining out now had to go somewhere else in my body. Because I had had so many lymph nodes removed, the lymph circulatory system was, in a sense, damaged and thus I was at risk for developing lymphedema. For some reason, I was petrified by the thought that I would end up with a swollen, painful upper arm. I obsessed about this daily, hourly. I won't scare you with either the statistics or the risks of lymphedema, but suffice it to say, it is not worth having. As it was, my underarm felt raw and swollen, and it was easy to imagine the lymphedema spreading. My imagination was running wild and I was sure that my arm was swelling up. I would check myself several times a day, and ask my husband to check me once more each evening to make sure that my arm was okay. I had been told that if you start to get lymphedema it is best treated immediately. I was determined to catch it at the start.

To help deal with potential lymphedema, and to head it off before it got started, I was referred to a physical therapist specializing in lymphatic massage. More than anything, the physical therapist gave me confidence that all was okay, and the strange sensations I was feeling in my underarm were actually related to the surgery and not to lymphedema. Thankfully, she too saw no signs of swelling. She gave me daily exercises to do and showed me how to do self-massage. I religiously followed her protocol for several months, until I got used to the new feeling in my upper arm and armpit, and my worries began to calm down. In addition, I did a series of ten lymphatic
massages. These massages are quite gentle and consist mainly of pushing on the affected areas, moving the lymphatic

fluid   into
alternate circulatory routes, away from the area that was
compromised by surgery. As my fears receded, I became less
obsessive about doing the self-massage and daily exercises.
Nowadays, I do a couple of exercises most days, and a couple
of times a week I do a self-massage. I get occasional blips on
the radar screen when I think something feels funny, and then I
usually talk to the physical therapist or go in for a massage.
This works at calming me down and certainly doesn't hurt. It
makes me feel like I am doing something good for myself, and
that too is a nice feeling.

TIPS FOR PREVENTING LYMPHEDEMA IN THE ARM:

1. Use your arm and hand a lot. In the beginning I was a bit afraid to carry things with my right hand, so I favored my left. Gradually I have returned to full use of my right arm, and I think that that is good for the lymphatic flow.

2. Exercise gently with weights. A few weeks after surgery I started lifting small hand weights to return both range of movement and strength to the area.

3. Get a compression stocking and glove for air travel. Because long-distance travel on airplanes can cause swelling, my physical therapist recommended using a sleeve and glove. Using it recently on my first plane trip since treatment made me remember how thankful I am that I don't have to wear one all the time. I found the glove very uncomfortable, switched to a gauntlet, and more recently used the stocking alone.

4. Know that after underarm surgery your underarm will feel funny. At first mine felt like I had a tennis ball in my armpit. After several weeks it shrank and became a golf ball. More than a year after surgery, I have now gotten used to this feeling – for the most part – but it is still not back to my pre-surgery state. This is the new normal.

5. Don't be afraid to ask your doctor, nurse, or physical therapist to check you out if you are worried that you may be developing lymphedema. It is far easier to solve the

problem when it is smaller, than when it has become a full-blown swelling.

My healing at home after surgery continued. It consisted of frequent naps, good food, and nice visitors. I found that I did not have much concentration for books or reading, which I normally love, and started watching mindless TV. After recuperating at home for about three weeks, I was ready for a change of scenery, and for me that meant going back to work. The pathology report was still not ready and treatment planning that would result was still looming on the horizon, as yet unsettled, but I was surprisingly patient. As the days turned into weeks, I began to prepare myself for the worst-case scenario— the dreaded chemo. I once again allowed the thought of it into my consciousness. In addition to emotionally preparing myself for the ordeal, I also began to introduce the very real possibility with my children. I told them that, while I had no new information, the way I figured, it was better to expect chemo and then be told that you would not need it, rather than the other way round. I convinced myself of this, too. I guess I do not like to be caught by surprise and this was my need for control taking over. I felt that rather than be caught unaware, I would be ready. I am sure that this is only one way to approach the unknown, but for me it worked, as I recognized once again how this was a situation where I virtually had no control. As the clock ticked, and we got closer to receiving the results from pathology, I had allowed chemo back onto my radar screen. This time I was scared but ready. Or so I thought.

Update #8 - August 6

This coming week I have a series of doctor appointments, and hope to find out what lays ahead for me— although, I have learned that at least for me, the best thing to do is take one day at a time, and not to assume that I actually will know by the end of the week. In terms of life lessons here, they go something like this:

- *no control*

- *no illusion of control*

- *don't even think that you have any control*

So if that is the case....I promise I will let you know when I know!

TIPS ON WAITING FOR RESULTS:

1. Take one day at a time.

2. Feel free to imagine all options, but don't allow yourself to obsess about the worst ones. When and if you do start to obsess tell yourself "stop." Sometimes that works.

3. Recognize that waiting is hard, and the limbo of not knowing can be more nerve-wracking than finally knowing – even if the results are less than positive.

4. Find five things to feel grateful for, no matter how big or small. (e.g. The sun is shining. I am going out to dinner tonight. I had a great walk this morning. etc. etc.)

5. Fill your time with people and activities that you enjoy. Spoil yourself. Now is the time.

[5]

To Know or Not To Know

'd like to take a break from my chronological journey now and embark on a few side trips, in order to share with you some features of my healing journey that were helpful to me. In this chapter we will consider the role of knowledge and information in healing, and in the following chapter we will spend some time with family and friends before returning to the chronological march of time.

I always considered myself a very curious person who wants to know everything there is to know. If you would have asked me to predict how much I would like to know about any disease I might have, I would have said, "Everything, of course." Interestingly, when I was an undergraduate completing my bachelor's degree, I wrote a seminar paper on how to tell a terminal patient that he was going to die. In that paper, I talked about the intricate dance between the terminal patient and his surroundings, and developed a model that explored the variations on the spectrum between knowing and not knowing, both on the part of the sick person and on the part of his caretakers and medical staff. The model looked at levels of disclosure, taking into account how open the patient was and how open the doctor was. There were four quadrants in this model. The two where the physician and patient were matched were: 1) open patient with disclosing doctor and 2) denying patient with non-disclosing doctor. The other two quadrants were mismatched: 3) denying patient with disclosing doctor and 4) open patient with non-disclosing doctor. Looking at the model today it seems simplistic and missing some very basic points, such as the place of family members. However the bottom line was that the first quadrant was the ideal and physicians should be open with their patients, who would then deal with their disease in a proactive way that to my mind was both desired and more rewarding. I had no doubts that I would want to know everything. Always. There was no question in my mind that if I was sick I would want to know all about what I had, the statistics, my odds of survival, and all that goes with total disclosure.

Thus, when after receiving my diagnosis of stage IIIA breast cancer I found myself avoiding the internet at all costs, I was frankly amazed. I could not believe it! I did NOT look up anything to do with breast cancer on the internet! Moreover, I did not read up on the statistics for my specific disease. I did not access any breast cancer sites on the internet and as a matter of fact, I stayed far away from anything to do with breast cancer on the internet including forums, blogs, and information sites. I did not even read any books on the subject. What a surprise to find myself in a situation where less was more and all I wanted to do was bury my head in the sand.

Why was I so avoidant? Why did I not want to learn everything there was to learn about my disease? Why was it that even the mere thought of reading an online article or book about breast cancer increased my anxiety tenfold? Was this something I should respect or fight? I was puzzled.

When taking a few moments to consider the situation, I realized that I was just barely hanging in there with what I knew about my disease and what my treatment plan would be. I felt that I had enough knowledge to make decisions and to keep a fairly even keel.   If I were to add to that additional reading about the full spectrum of possibilities, or about other women's experiences, I thought that I would likely start to feel overwhelmed and sink into a negative run of thoughts. So being avoidant was a self-protecting move. In general, I am a very suggestible person.   This attribute can be very helpful when doing self-hypnosis or guided imagery. The flip side of suggestibility is that every time I heard about something related to MY disease, I immediately imagined myself with the new symptom or ailment. Understanding this about myself reassured me that it was really okay not to seek out information about my disease.   My avoidance was so great that for weeks after my surgery I did not even read my own pathology report. Several days had gone by after receiving the report when I asked my husband to read it and to report back to me with the highlights. Interestingly, it even took him a few weeks to get around to reading it. It seems to me that avoidance and denial have some mighty fine aspects to them. This includes the ability to continue to live life without feeling too scared or too overwhelmed by insurmountable odds.   After all, even if the odds are against you, each person is a sample of one, and if you beat the odds you have beat them by 100%. This goes along with the old adage of why worry about the things that you cannot change. I felt that my diagnosis was something I could not change, and I was happy to reduce worry. By reducing information overload (a common condition in our electronic age), I was able to reduce unhelpful worry.

The fact that I found denial and avoidance so helpful in my new condition actually came into conflict on occasion with the medical professionals I was dealing with. My oncologist had told me at our first meeting that he was a "straight shooter" and that he would always tell me the truth. Initially, that made me very happy and was, in fact, one of the reasons why I had chosen him to be my doctor. It suited my beliefs about myself and what I was sure I would want; it suited my abhorrence of subterfuge and lies. Well, cancer has a way of turning things upside down, and over the months of treatment the oncologist's straightforwardness and honesty was not always exactly what I needed. As I moved into the world of cancer, things were changing and sometimes I found his approach a bit too jarring.

One example that comes to mind is when I consulted with the

oncologist about the extent of my second surgery. Since the pathology results from my initial surgery had come back with the finding that the margins of the tumor were not clean, it was clear that I would need to do a second surgery. The question was, once again: lumpectomy or mastectomy. The surgeon told me that it didn't much matter what kind of surgery I had – lumpectomy or mastectomy – since, to his mind, my life expectancy would be the same, or similar, with either scenario. The real concern, he reminded me (and this is the part that I wish he would have skipped), was the ever-present threat of metastases, since seven out of the twenty-two lymph nodes that had been removed were cancerous. This, he said, was just to put things into perspective for me so I would not obsess so much about making the surgery decision. Was this the perspective I needed? Did I want to hear this now? On some level, I appreciated his honesty and knew that what he said was true. On the other hand, his saying this created a new reality for me that was frightening. With the perspective of a year, I can see myself in that third quadrant of patient who doesn't want to know, paired with the doctor who tells everything. Yes, this is a mismatch, and even if the mismatch is temporary, it sure can cause pain.

As the months rolled on and breast cancer settled into a more permanent part of my self-image, my resistance to outside information lowered a bit, and I would occasionally make forays out to gather information on very specific topics. For example, I was very interested in diet and cancer and, in particular, whether eating soy was beneficial or detrimental, since I was diagnosed with estrogen-positive cancer. I did a search on that and found some very useful information. Another search I did was on alcohol and breast cancer. I love a glass of wine or beer and the thought that I would have to give it up forever was actually painful. Through my search I was able to learn more and, while I am still not entirely clear on it, I tend to go with my doctor's advice: A glass of wine is fine on one condition – that it is good wine!

As a rule, I was still very careful with internet access because I found that there was so much information and misinformation on the net that surfing could be a dangerous pastime. However, toward the end of my treatment year, I signed on to a couple of website forums. There I found communities of women very actively engaged in discussion and eager to help one another. On the one hand, this was very helpful. If I wanted to find out the connection between Tamoxifen (a medicine I was taking to reduce the absorption of estrogens) and yeast infections, the answer was there. If I wanted to kvetch, there were people willing to listen. On the other hand, I ran the risk of misinformation and, even scarier to me was hearing stories of women with breast cancer who were

not   beating   the
disease.   By its very nature, the internet provides access to huge numbers of people at any given time. If the cure rate in breast cancer these days is about 80% that means that 20% are going in the wrong direction. Many of them are on the internet and, by hanging out there, I had to face the very real evidence and scary possibility that I, too, could be one of the 20%. Most of the time, I could convince myself that the odds were good, and I could carry on and live without a dark cloud hanging over my head. However, when my internet buddies were getting sick and dying, that was too close to home and too hard for me. I did not want to face that stark possibility.

In recent months, I think that I have found a reasonably happy medium between feast and famine. There are two websites that I access when I need information about something related to breast cancer. I find that it is good for me to know that they are there if I should need them. However, on a day-to-day basis I stay reasonably far away from the sites and their forums because I find that they take both a lot of time and a lot of emotional energy that I prefer to spend elsewhere.

Having said all that, I know that there are many people who find a great deal of support through online forums, which has made all the difference in their healing.   I think that this is a good   time   to reiterate and recognize once again the differences among us. Each and every one of us is unique with our own personality, our own likes and dislikes, our own ways of meeting the world, and our own support systems.   What worked for me may or may not be the right thing for you or your loved one. What I would urge you to do is to take a moment to check in with yourself and where you are; acknowledge that it may be perfectly okay to moderate your internet diet. You may want to know everything there is about your disease. But, you may prefer not to. You may be surprised at your answers. Remember: there is not a right or wrong here. Be prepared to feel one way this week or month, and then change your mind farther down the road. Be open to the possibility of that change. What is right for you is right for you, and don't let anyone tell you otherwise.

The interesting thing for me was how surprised I was by my behavior. If you had asked me a year ago how I would react to having cancer, my prediction would have been 100% wrong. But when I was ill, I found that this balance between knowing and not knowing was right for me. I listened inward and was much happier for that.

Cancer Resources on the Internet

Despite everything I have written above, I want to share with you an annotated short list of some links that I found helpful:

1. <u>The Crazy Sexy Breast Cancer Group</u>

This is a group on Kris Carr's site. The Crazy Sexy Life site is geared to healthful living in general, and there are many group boards within that site dedicated to specific health issues including several for women with breast cancer. I found the cancer groups to be particularly supportive, gentle and friendly.

http://my.crazysexylife.com/group/crazysexybreastcancer

2. <u>The American Cancer Society Discussion Boards</u>

The American Cancer Society has a discussion board for every type of cancer imaginable. I found the breast cancer site helpful with very specific information, but did not spend much time hanging out there. From what I could tell, the site was friendly and supportive as well.

http://csn.cancer.org/forum

3 .I also followed two blogs of woman who were dealing with different kinds of cancer. I found their writings interesting and helpful. I am not including their URLs because these types of blogs come and go, and addresses change frequently. I suggest that you do an internet search for blogs of women with breast cancer if you are interested.

TIPS ON LEARNING ABOUT YOUR CANCER:

1. Find reliable sources of information. Don't assume that because something is on the internet it is reliable.

2. Decide how much you want to know, and don't let anybody tell you otherwise. This is a personal decision, and yours and only yours to make.

3. Allow people in your environment that same amount of freedom to determine what the right level of information is for them.

4. Be assertive with friends or family who are sharing information you are not interested in. For example, you may not want to hear about Great Aunt Rose who had a cancer just like yours. Feel free to tell them you don't wish to discuss this.

5. Remember: you don't HAVE to know everything. You can choose how much and what you want to know, and ask others to respect   your   wishes.

[6]

Family and Friends

One more side trip that we will take before entering the world of chemo is to the world of family and friends, who form the cornerstone of any healing program. A theme running through this book has been their ever-present support. It is worth spending more than a few moments on this topic because, while common wisdom tells us how important family and friends are, this is strongly backed up by extensive psychological research which shows that the single most important factor in an individual's resilience is the amount of social support he or she has. For me that has certainly been true.

It might be interesting to take a moment to do an exercise together that will help us look at our social supports. One easy way to do this is to take a blank sheet of paper and a pencil or pen and draw a big spider web. Now do the following:

1. Place yourself at the center of the web.

2. Now fill in a person's name at every junction of the web. The first ring of the web, closest to you, should be populated with the names of people with whom you have daily or almost-daily contact (it may be a phone call, email or even a thought – the contact doesn't have to be live and in person). This first ring

of the web may include your spouse, children, parents, best friends and the like.

3. In the second ring of the web you can place people with whom you are in contact, but perhaps weekly. This circle might include

co-workers, good friends, and other family members.

4. On the outer rings of the web you will place people with whom you have occasional contact, such as neighbors, more distant

relatives, co-workers, friends, community members, facebook or internet forum friends.

5. You can also use the web to describe the quality of the relationship. A dotted line can indicate a tenuous relationship. A strong line might indicate a very intense relationship. Be creative.

This exercise is a very dynamic piece of work, but it will give you a picture of where you are right now. It can also help you gain perspective on relationships that exist, that are in trouble, or that are missing. You may find that people have moved from one ring to the other during your cancer journey.   Many of us have   been disappeared by close friends who "disappeared" on us during the months of treatment. These may have been balanced by friends who surprised us with their warmth, kindness and readiness to help. Life is dynamic, and nothing is more so than our web of relationships.

Upon examination, my closest circle was my immediate family, including both husband and children. They stepped up to the plate in a way that, to my mind, was remarkable even while being expected. They were there when I needed and wanted them, without hovering. If I wanted to go out for lunch or a short drive, they were available and made time for me. I felt that I was a priority in this year of their lives, and all I had to do was open my mouth and they would come running. It was actually quite nice! This is an interesting state of affairs, particularly with teens and young adults, who are so often eager to find the right distance and level of independence from Mom and Dad. But the year of my cancer journey was different. I had the feeling that my children were like little puppy dogs who needed to come back to be close to Mom, to touch base and make sure I was okay. I loved the frequent visits, the phone calls, the spontaneous dates, and their willingness to make personal sacrifices in order to spend family time together, without the usual grumbling or difficulties in scheduling. The alacrity with which they were willing to drop everything was sometimes even a little scary.

While cancer never chooses a fortuitous time to rear its ugly head, for our 23-year-old son Shuey (a nickname for Yehoshua), the timing was particularly inauspicious, as he was due to set out on a long–awaited trek to Africa. Many young Israelis, upon completing compulsory three-year army service, choose to make a trip to some exotic location for a period of several months to a year. Shuey had long ago chosen Africa as his destination and for the last half year had been eagerly planning his adventure and working hard to save money for the trip. Tickets had been ordered and paid for and the departure date marked on the calendar several months before my cancer diagnosis. He was due to set out about six weeks after I got the grim news. When I was diagnosed, the question came up whether he should take his trip. I was determined that he depart for his journey as planned and not make any modifications because of me. After all, how could he help out in this situation? What could he really do? At this point in time before surgery and possibly chemo or radiation, I was feeling okay, and continuing with my life as much as possible, which included going to work and social events, taking care of the household and family, as well as following through with the additional burden of many doctor visits and diagnostic tests. I didn't need any particular help from him and when I saw the hesitation in his eyes, I urged him to go. Shuey was due to leave about one week post-surgery, before the pathology report was due and before we had a decision about the rest of treatment. I encouraged him to proceed as planned and promised him that I would be in regular contact and be totally up front with him, telling him everything that was going on. I was hoping that this would both encourage him and help him deal with an imagination that might run wild at such a distance. I knew that if he hung around, he wouldn't have much to do and it would be a very big disappointment to him.

I recognized that despite my encouragement, it was very difficult for him to leave at this time and so, to help ease his conscience, I told him how much I would enjoy traveling vicariously with him. I have always wanted to travel the world and toyed with the idea of writing a travel blog. I thought that some armchair travel to Africa would be just the thing to help me escape my narrow world of cancer. Little did I know how true this was. I decided to write a blog about Shuey's travels, which would allow me to learn about all the places he was traveling to, immerse myself in his trip, and share it with friends and family. But there was a twist. Since my son is not one of the biggest communicators and I really had no idea what he was doing, I quickly decided that my blog would work on the theory of suppositions rather than waiting to hear exactly what he had done or where he had gone. The way it worked was that Shuey would tell me the name of the place he was visiting and occasionally even what he was planning to do over the next couple of days. I would scour the internet for information and pictures about the area and then write a blog reporting on what I imagined he was doing, complete with pictures of the various locations. For example, one day he told me that he would be in the area of Lake Naivasha in Kenya. After spending not a small amount of time reading up on the area and looking at photos on the web, I decided that Shuey would likely choose to go biking in Hell's Gate National Park through the lush and verdant countryside. I had no idea if he really was going to do this but I thought that it might be a nice adventure, so I blogged his recent doings and location along with a picture of tourists biking through the park. With tongue in cheek I wrote that he was the third from the left in the blue shirt. When he got to the internet and checked the blog, he told me that I was right on that time, only his shirt was red! If you are so inclined, you can check out the blog at www.naomibaum.wordpress.com. I thoroughly enjoyed vicariously visiting the locations Shuey had chosen, and looking at the pictures of magnificent scenery that he was most probably enjoying along with me. Our family avidly read the blog and, while I might not have been 100% accurate as to Shuey's exploits, we were able to track the general direction of his adventures, and I certainly had a blast doing it.

The blog allowed me to escape my current situation and distract myself during the long weeks after chemo. Climbing Mt. Kenya and reaching the peak was one of the high points of my adventure,
particularly when I found a YouTube video that documented it. Armchair travel through the internet was the only way that I would be traveling this year, and I was making the most of it. When my son returned from his trip, I felt that I knew where he had been, and at least some of the things he had experienced.

The role of fantasy in healing cancer should not be underestimated.

For me, surrounded by family and friends, it is hard to imagine facing cancer alone and without extensive social supports. However, every person's situation in life is different. Some of us have many family members who live in close proximity.   Others   have   only occasional contact with far-flung family, and their close circles consist of friends and co-workers. For those who do not have ready-made, built-in supports, cancer may be a particularly trying time. Reaching out to community supports, to internet friends, or dusting off some forgotten relationships may be helpful at a time like this.

My second web of support consisted of parents and in-laws, brothers and sisters, and several close friends. Their phone calls, visits, concern, and eagerness to spend time with us was both
touching and supportive. The physical help of food preparation, Mom's chicken soup after chemo, and everyone's moral support were invaluable.

Work colleagues, neighbors, friends and extended family rounded out my outer circles of support. People in these circles often called, wrote, and inquired how they could help. Fortunately, I did not need a lot of extra help so, even though the offers were heartfelt, I didn't often accept them. While I did learn to ask for what I needed, a bit more than I had in the past, this was still a difficult thing to do. Having spent most of my life on the giving end rather than the receiving end, I found the switch in roles both disconcerting and difficult to get used to.

One of my clearest memories from my pre-chemo session with the nurse who was preparing me for what to expect, was her telling me that I would have to get used to asking for and accepting help. She assured me that it would not be easy, but that I should try to get used to it. In reality, what happened was that many, many people asked if they could help, but their question was such a general one that I found it difficult to answer. On the other hand, if somebody called me with a specific offer, such as, "Can I bring over a meal? Or a pot of soup?" I almost invariably said yes, and was truly grateful. This was a good lesson for me for the future. Would I remember this when I was once again on the giving end and not the receiving end? At some point during the year I actually became annoyed by the vague offers for help. The people who said, "How can I help you?" or "If there is anything you need..." were well-meaning but irksome. I certainly wasn't going to ASK for food. I was not desperate and we were managing. But when specific offers did come along, I found that they were a big help, physically, and probably even more important, emotionally. Getting a plate of muffins or a tray of chicken felt like a big warm hug and gave me a lift.

Relating to this outer circle was tricky. I believe that people really did care when they thought about me and what I was going through, but I was not at the top of their list of priorities, and that was actually okay. A friendly hello, a hug, a heartfelt "how are you?" can go a long way.

Now what about the disappointments? Those people you were counting on who have fizzled or haven't come through for you. What can you do? It is certainly hard to have any perspective during this time and, although the only thing that stars center stage for us this year is cancer with a capital C, others around us are trying to live their lives, go to work, and carry on. Having a conversation and laying out our expectations can be a helpful start to repairing misunderstandings, but this is not always easy to do. People in our outer circles who have disappointed or let us down may be best left alone and avoided during this trying time. It is possible to repair these relationships when you are feeling stronger and can recognize that for some people illness is very confusing, scary. Right now you might decide not be around people like that. This is a year to choose your friends, and feel comfortable saying no to those you would rather not spend time with.

Below are some tips that may help you navigate through this difficult time.

TIPS ON GETTING AND GIVING HELP:

1. Sit down and make a very specific list of all the areas in which you would like help.

2. Appoint someone close to you (a friend or family member) to help you, a "gatekeeper" of sorts. This person can help you make the list of what you need. Examples of areas you might want help with include: dealing with medical/insurance bureaucracy and paperwork, household help, cooking, babysitting, shopping or transportation.

3. If it is hard for you to ask for help when someone says the invariable, "if you need anything just call, " forward all offers of help to your gatekeeper. For example, if your neighbor asks, "How can I help?" you can just tell her to call "X" who is keeping an organized list of what you need and who's doing what.

4. Remember that most people like to help. It makes them feel better and more in control in a situation (cancer) that is out of their control and therefore quite scary. Consider that you are doing the helpers a favor by giving them a specific task.

5. The more direction you can give people, the better. Very few people out there are mind

readers. This goes for people who are closest to you as well. They too need direction. So don't be afraid to ask for what you need.

6. If you are a friend or family member of the person with cancer and on the giving end, suggest something specific that you could do: driving to chemo, a cooked meal, taking over a carpool shift, picking up groceries, babysitting, a day out. Vague offers of "if you need help let me know," become annoying after a while and may seem insincere.

[7]

Talking Cancer

One of the big lessons I learned during my year of cancer had to do with communication. I have already spent a fair amount of time talking about how to tell people you have cancer. The question is: how much to tell and to whom? Additionally, once friends and family know you have cancer – what are the expectations? Do you have to tell everybody everything? With whom do you share on a regular basis? And how much do you tell?

As I reflect upon these questions now, several months after completing treatment, I am struck by the fact that while I was very open, and wanted to share just about everything that was going on with my innermost circle or family and friends, when people from what I perceived to be more outer circles of my web asked intimate questions, I felt intruded upon. I resented their questions and I shut down. While I knew at the time that their intentions were good and heartfelt, there was a mismatch between what they were asking and what I wanted to share. I think that this mismatch between visitor and visitee happens more often than we might think. The following story will illustrate that point.

One of the many things that is surprising about cancer is who pops out of the woodwork and takes a personal interest in you, and how they do it. There were good souls who quietly brought over food without a lot of fanfare, warming my heart with their caring. There were others who called or sent an e-mail or text message wishing me well and making me feel good that they took the time to let me know that they were thinking about me. Some folks called and asked if it would be convenient to visit, and others just showed up when it was convenient for them. Sometimes that was welcome, and at other times it just wasn't. What to do with that scenario? Picture it: you are just getting ready to lie down and take a nap. You are feeling cranky and blue. You want to be alone, and the doorbell rings with an unannounced visitor. What to do?

A person going through cancer treatment needs to develop the ability to clearly state what she needs or wants at any given time. If the visit is inconvenient, now is the time to develop assertiveness skills and say, "Thanks for coming by, but I was just going to lay down for a nap." If you don't want to talk on the phone, you are allowed to say that this is an inconvenient time for you. Entertaining visitors can be very tiring, and you must remember that your first priority is to yourself. Even if you have been a "pleaser" all your life, this is the time to change. Ask yourself: What do YOU need right now? What do you WANT right now?

I recall particularly clearly a visit from a casual friend when I was recuperating from surgery. She had dropped in unannounced and as we sat in my kitchen drinking tea, she began asking all sorts of questions about my surgery, diagnosis and treatment plan. I duly, albeit tiredly, answered each question even though I felt that they were invasive, and went beyond the bounds of our superficial relationship. After about ten minutes of this back and forth she suddenly looked me straight in the face and asked, "Are you worried?" The question floored me. I felt that my private space was being invaded and I did not welcome the question. Of course I was worried! What did she think? Certainly thoughts of death and mortality were keeping me up at nights! Yes, some nights I woke up in a cold sweat and couldn't breathe, picturing myself suffocating in a grave. Did I want to share this with her? NO. NO. NO. As a matter of fact, I found the question both insensitive and presumptuous. This visitor was not a close friend, not somebody with whom I chose to share my deepest thoughts, concerns and fears. Now she clearly felt like an intruder. Thinking this over later I thought to myself that I could have stopped her line of questioning much earlier by saying, "Let's talk about something else." Instead, I dutifully answered, getting more and more annoyed on the inside. When she asked about worries, I quickly ended the visit. I stood up and said sarcastically, "Worries? Nah! What's there to be worried about?" She looked startled. I continued, "By the way, I need to go and get dinner ready now, so I am sorry to have to shoo you out." And off she went, much to my relief. No matter how many times I tried to tell myself this friend was a kind person who made the effort to visit me, every time I thought of her visit I felt my heart beating faster and the anger rising in my gorge.

I have turned this conversation over in my mind again and again, wondering what upset me so much about it. Worries were not new to me. She was not creating fears that did not exist. She was merely reminding me of them. For me, the conversation both presumed too much intimacy and was intrusive. I was upset that I had not asserted myself a bit earlier and shooed her out before that question came up. On the other hand, I knew she only meant well. She had taken time out of her busy schedule to sit with me and try to cheer me on. Unfortunately, her visit had the opposite effect.

I have since realized that many of us do not know how to be with a sick person. What is helpful? What to do? What to say? When to say it? Who should take the lead?

I came across a very lovely piece on the internet by Mary Beth
Williams, a fellow sojourner on the cancer journey, about how to talk with friends and family about cancer that speaks to this point. I have liberally modified her list, but the inspiration came directly from her and helped me realize that this is an issue not only for me, but for many of us on the cancer path. As you read these rules that I have liberally adapted, remember – this is meant for friends or family members of the cancer patient, and spoken directly from the mouth of someone who has cancer.

TIPS ON HOW TO TALK WITH CANCER PATIENTS:

When visiting with cancer patients keep these rules in mind.

1. This is about the person with cancer, not about you.

Cancer makes everybody nervous. "If she could get cancer, so could I." But remember when you speak to the cancer patient: it is not their job to make you feel better or allay your fears. They have enough of their own and don't need yours.

2. This is a very bad time to disappear.

It doesn't take big gestures. It takes less than a minute to send an email or a text or pick up the phone or walk over to someone in the supermarket and say, "How are you?" That's all it takes to let someone know you're still on their team. And that minute can be the difference between   a miserable, scary day and feeling supported and reassured.

3. Don't blame the victim.

I don't know anyone with cancer who hasn't heard a version of, "Did you smoke? Did you sunbathe? What happened?" To people with cancer this sounds an awful lot like, "Tell me how you screwed up so I won't make the same mistake." Similarly, don't bother telling them about how stress, lifestyle or bad thoughts cause cancer, or how a positive attitude will cure cancer.

4. Don't be hasty with the best-case scenarios.

People with cancer appreciate your encouragement. However, they don't need someone making sweeping pronouncements about the future. They might not appreciate your vision that "we" will "battle" this. And if the prognosis is bad, cancer patients don't want you to tell them that no, it's not. Here's the thing about cancer – some of us are going to die, not because we're quitters, but because that's how it works. If someone with cancer is telling you that, shut up and listen.

5. Don't rush the cure.

Even if things are going well, let it go at its own pace. I can't count the number of times people have called me a "survivor" or said things like, "So, are you cured?" This happens a lot to those of us in the club. It makes us feel a little rushed here. Like you're eager to wrap this thing up and move on already so that you can forget about it.

7. Don't be a downer.

You don't need to quote harrowing statistics right now, or mention your neighbor who was in so much pain at the end. Being sympathetic does not mean telling people that you don't know how they're possibly coping right now (hint: they don't have a choice), or what a grueling ordeal it all must be.

8. Be guided by the person's cues.

Some people will post status updates on facebook from their chemo treatments. Others will prefer not to talk about it. Respect their limits — it's their cancer party, and they get to call the cancer shots. You don't have to cure anybody. You don't have to cheerlead. You don't have to do very much at all. Just be a friend. Stick around. Let them know they are not forgotten even if they're not around as much lately. They are not scary because they look different. And reassure them that if they can handle this, you can love them enough to handle this too.

[8]

Preparing for Chemo

Update #9 - August 12

I continue to heal from surgery, and am definitely getting back to myself. This week I actually went to work for a couple of hours. But time marches on, and the path report has come in leading me to the news: this coming week I will start chemo, every other week for 16 weeks. The protocol is called ACT-dense dose. Three different drugs are used – two of them for weeks 1-8, and the third for weeks 9-16. The treatment is given every other week, in the day oncology unit at Sha'arei Zedek Medical Center.

Chemo for many people is the watershed that determines how serious their cancer is. Up until the time I realized that I was to have chemo, I was able to live with the illusion that my cancer was discovered "early" in the game and was not too lethal. I was pretty sure that I would recover well. But the moment I heard that I would need chemo, that house of cards tumbled, and I was forced to acknowledge that what I had was actually serious. My cancer had progressed into the lymph nodes and was not at an early stage. In fact, my pathology report indicated that seven out of twenty-two lymph nodes were cancerous and that put me at Stage IIIA, a clear indication for chemotherapy, which can itself be life-threatening.

I received the news about chemo sitting in my oncologist's office about three weeks after surgery. I can recall every detail of that fateful meeting. He was facing the computer looking for my

pathology report, and it was taking what seemed to be an interminably long time for him to find them. As he fiddled with the computer, my anxiety grew. At some point I said, "Doctor, I am getting pretty anxious here." He turned his head, looked me in the eye and said, "Anxious? About what?" I answered without missing a beat, "About the little things like do I need chemo? Will I die?"

Turning in his chair to face me directly he said, "Chemo? That's a no brainer. Of course you need chemo. Will you die from this cancer? I do not know. I will, however, do my best to keep you alive. That's my job. But there are no guarantees."

Talk about a cold shower. My immediate reaction to this brief

exchange was an internal voice that piped up inside of me, asking: "How do I know this guy is a real doctor? Maybe he is a charlatan or a quack? And, come to think of it, where are all his diplomas?" I scanned the bare walls of the office. Not a diploma or certificate in sight. I instantly flashed to the television show I grew up on, 60 Minutes, a documentary expose show. I'd once seen an episode that uncovered imposters who were fraudulently running hospital departments with no medical training. I thought, "Maybe this guy is one of them!" Without missing a beat I asked the doctor, who had turned back to the computer, "Where are your diplomas?"

"What do I need diplomas for?" Now I knew he was a fraud, and for sure I wouldn't need chemo. I answered more diplomatically than I felt, "How can I know what medical school you went to if your diplomas are not on the wall?"

"Remember. I told you that you can ask me anything. Anything at all."

"Ok. So where did you go to medical school?" "University of Pennsylvania."

Bingo. That was where my husband, who had been sitting beside me quietly during this peculiar interchange, had attended medical school more than thirty years ago. It is a leading medical school in the United States. You have to be pretty damned smart to get in to Penn, and to complete the four years of study. The rest of the meeting was taken up by my husband and my physician exchanging medical school anecdotes and reminiscing about long-gone

professors, as I quietly sat there, trying to absorb the knowledge that I really would be starting chemo within a week. Thankfully, I was now reassured that the physician sitting in front of me who would be running my "show" was a well-trained, professional doctor.

Yet no matter how much you think you are ready to hear the word "chemo", actually hearing it was pretty scary indeed. I could barely absorb the information the doctor gave me about the type of chemo I would undergo, never mind the more technical aspects regarding which day, and what the next steps were. It was very good that I had my husband with me at that appointment. He could hear more clearly what the doctor was saying. This way, later in the day, we could review the details that had escaped me, and have a chance to process with each other what had been said.

Now, after waiting patiently over the course of weeks and months for the results of diagnostic tests and pathology reports, all of a sudden things were moving quickly. Very quickly. Too quickly. I was scheduled to start chemo almost immediately. Up until this moment it seemed like nobody was too concerned and we had all the time in the world. Now it appeared, things were urgent. Very urgent. Apparently, there was no good reason to wait and every reason in the world to get started immediately. This urgency was scary as well.

Side Effects: The Whole Nine Yards

Before chemo could begin, I had one more appointment. I was directed to schedule a session with the breast cancer nurse to prepare me for what lay ahead. Of all my medical contacts, appointments and meetings, and there were many, that one meeting that prepared me for chemo was to my mind singularly helpful and supportive. Susan, the nurse was very open and generous with her time, and we had a very long, frank conversation covering all pertinent points, preparing me for what I might expect both physically and emotionally. There is often a very fine line between scaring people with possible side effects and preparing them appropriately. This experienced nurse walked the line with grace. She was supportive without being mushy, informative without being overwhelming and practical without being bossy. She talked about losing my hair and getting fitted for a wig, the possibility of mouth sores and how to prevent them by rinsing with baking soda, sex during chemo (recommended), and asking for and receiving help from neighbors and friends. Most importantly, she left the door open for further questions and remained accessible throughout the duration of my treatment.

Volumes have been written detailing the horrors of chemo and the numerous side effects, ranging from the physical to emotional. I found that while it was helpful for me to know that whatever side effect I was having was normal, there was a law of diminishing returns when it came to self-education. As a highly suggestible person, I found that if I read or heard about a symptom, I started worrying about it and then imagining that I might have it. If I didn't know about it, then I didn't worry about it until it actually showed up. The balance between educating one's self and scaring one's self is often a fine line. Clearly, every cancer patient needs to figure out what is right for them. After trial and error, I found that what worked for me was to get a general overview of what to expect without too many details about the possible side effects. When prepared accordingly, I felt prepared without opening the door to my tendency to hypochondria.

So let's talk about some of the side effects, beginning with hair loss. Of all the chemo side effects that people "on the outside" seem to be aware of (now that I had taken the big step over to the land of chemo I viewed myself as a cancer "insider"), hair loss seems to take center stage, perhaps because this is the most obvious side effect. You just can't *not notice* a bald person. As I mentioned, the chemo prep nurse had encouraged me to get fitted for a wig to help prepare for my certain hair loss, considering the cocktail of drugs that I would be taking. I dutifully did what I was told and rushed to the wig store while I still had my hair, so that I could get something that would look more or less like the me I knew and was comfortable with.   It is interesting to me that some people take this time as an

opportunity to try out new hairstyles and colors. I was less daring at first, and purchased a wig that was short, brown and curly, just like my own hair. I never wore it. In addition to the wig, I went out and splurged on several colorful scarves.

After making my purchases in preparation for the hair loss that was supposed to occur sometime after the second treatment, I decided to take matters back into my own hands as best I could, in yet another bid for control over this new and scary terrain. I had seen countless movies with heart-rending scenes in which the heroine's hair is falling out in chunks and she is looking into the mirror at herself and crying hysterically. I definitely did not want that! So, rather than waiting for the inevitable to happen, I decided to do a pre-emptive "buzz" cut and shave my hair down to a very close, military crew. While a buzz cut is fairly dramatic and does call attention to one's self, it is one step before bald, and I thought that it would give both me and the people around me time to get used to my new look. By courageously (and it did take courage) deciding to go all the way rather than waiting for my hair to start falling out in clumps, I was retrieving a small but important feeling of control over my life at a point in time when it felt like everything was spinning wildly out of control. Choosing when and how to cut my hair may   seem inconsequential but it was huge.

My perceptive family decided to make an event out of my haircut. The kids organized a pre-chemo party in which the high point would be my haircut. My eldest son, Eitan, had become skilled at giving haircuts to friends and neighbors (mostly male) over the last ten years and I was trusting that he would do a good job. It certainly beat going to the local barber. All of my children and grandchildren, as well as my husband, assembled in the late afternoon as the sun was beginning to set. Didi and Smadar hosted the event at their home in a rural community not far from the sea. The grills were heating up as I sat down for my haircut. Each one of my kids took a ceremonial snip of my dark (dyed) curls, and then my barber son cleaned up and finished the cut. I went to the bathroom to shower and survey the effects. Not too bad. Actually, not bad at all. I could get used to this! It certainly felt great, and cool – in more ways than one.

In an amazing gesture of support, my youngest daughter, Shlomzion, decided to shave her head as well. She looked absolutely gorgeous. Having her go through the haircut with me was a remarkable experience. I felt, at least in this, I was not alone. My confidence was bolstered by having someone along with me, experiencing the comments, the reactions and the cool breezes on our scalps. I still would have a few weeks to enjoy my new look before my shorn locks would disappear completely. Shlomzion and I have always looked alike, and now with the haircuts the similarity was even more pronounced. Looking at her and seeing how good she looked, I was reassured that I looked okay. After we both finished our haircut, several of my grandsons and my husband decided to go along for the ride, and they also got buzz cuts. Although their cuts were less dramatic, nevertheless their gestures were heartwarming. It was a haircut fest!

After the haircuts were finished we settled down to a barbecue feast, family talk and then a round of blessings, and gifts. I felt like the birthday girl, and it wasn't even my birthday. The most moving part of the evening for me was when Eitan (the barber) read a prayer he had composed that morning to accompany my journey of chemo. His opening words were borrowed from the Traveler's Prayer that is part of the Jewish prayer book, and they brought tears to my eyes. He had successfully incorporated all aspects of this terrible journey I was embarking on: my fears and questions, the family and friends who surrounded me, the physicians and nurses who were working hard to heal me, and my faith in God, the greatest Healer of all. He had written an incredible prayer. I planned to say it the very next morning before the medicines began coursing through my veins. Since that time I have shared the prayer with thousands, both via the internet, and on cards that I printed up and distributed in hospitals in Israel and abroad. Eitan's prayer sounds a resonant chord in everyone who reads it and has brought succor to many. That evening with my children by my side filled me with love and gratefulness and prepared me, I hoped, for the auspicious day ahead.

Wayfarers' Prayer

upon Embarking on the Journey of Healing

May it be Your will, merciful and healing Father, to lead me on this journey in peace, to accompany me in peace, to stand by my side and to give me life, health, happiness and peace.

Give me the strength to bear this cancer with dignity, and the power to endure it and be healed.

Protect me from pain, sadness and despair, and from all the discomforts that are drawing near.

Send skill, wisdom and understanding to my doctors and nurses, Your faithful messengers, to sow goodness and light in my body.

Help the chemicals accurately do their work, rooting out disease and bringing compassion to the healthy parts of my body, making room for the good to strengthen and take root.

Wrap me in goodness so that I will be strong of body and spirit, to live a good, full life. Give me the strength to traverse this difficult period with joy and faith - with a closeness to You.

Help me stay mindful of my family and friends who are walking this road with me, and who, with me, raise their eyes to You, Knower of all mysteries.

"The mouth that decrees is the mouth that pardons." "Because You are the source of all, and from Your hand comes that which we return to You." "The afflicted pray for Your embrace and pour out their hearts before Hashem."

All-high, awesome G-d, I stand before you as a vessel full of submission and fear. I do not understand why I have become sick, but I understand that it is Your will.

Grant me the strength to receive Your will with love, and show me the way to find grace, favor, kindness and mercy in Your eyes.

"G-d created a pure heart for me and instilled within me a new spirit."

Bring me speedily to a great light. G-d's salvation can come in a moment. Let all disease and evil transform - in the blink of an eye - into goodness and blessings for me and for all Israel, as it is written: "And Hashem your G-d will transform the curse into a blessing, because Hashem your G-d loves you."

Because You hear the prayer of each person. Blessed are You, who hears prayer. May the words of my mouth and the meditations of my heart be acceptable before You, Hashem, my Rock and Redeemer.

A printable copy of this prayer in both Hebrew and English can be found online at www.naomibaum.com.

Tips on Preparing for Chemo:

1. Decide how you will handle potential hair loss and explore options of wigs, hair implants, scarves and hats. This will help you feel ready for what is to come.

2. Organize your household, keeping in mind that you may not be feeling well for several days or more after the chemo. Plan for backup for your household roles, whether they be cooking, childcare, paperwork, cleaning or something else.

3. Prepare your co-workers and arrange, if possible, to have someone pick up your slack at work.

4. Much of what will happen you cannot prepare for. After you have done what you can, try to live one day at a time (easier said than done, but it is always good to have something to aspire to!).

5. Allow your friends and family to spoil you.

6. Spoil yourself.

[9]

Chemo

Update #10 – August 19

Hi all,

So the good news is that I started my chemo treatment (ACT-dense dose – and I now know what each letter stands for – you can test me!) yesterday, and it is today, and I am feeling ok. Pretty good, actually. I have been trying to find words all day to describe the new sensations my body is experiencing, and it is a challenge. Yesterday I actually felt that my body was at war with itself. It was a most uncomfortable, confusing feeling. It was almost like the forces of good and evil struggling inside of me. As I think about it now, several Harry Potter scenes come to mind.

The first day of chemo dawned bright and hot in late August. I decided to mark the occasion, by wearing a new blouse I had recently bought, and reciting the "Shehechiyanu" blessing, "Blessed are You, King of the Universe, Who has kept me alive and brought me to this day." I had said this blessing since childhood every time I wore a new article of clothing or ate a new fruit, and on the eve of each holiday. Now this blessing took on special meaning for me and I created opportunities to say it as often as I could, concentrating on every word. I focused on feeling grateful and blessed that I lived in a time and place when chemo was readily available, and there were ways to treat this insidious disease. This was a gift I gave myself. That is not to say that I didn't occasionally slip into self-pity, because I certainly did. When I was feeling sorry for myself I cried and felt isolated, alone, and bummed out. I did not like that feeling at all. It did not feel helpful. It did not feel healing. I did not feel that I was "getting it all out". My tears were not cleansing. I actually found that I, who often cry at the drop of a hat, intensely disliked crying for myself now.

So what did I do when I wasn't feeling so grateful, but focused on being alone in the world with this HUGE cancer that is attacking my body, and the scary possibility that I may not make it? There are no easy tricks here, and no magic pills. Sometimes I was able to give myself a mental shake or a kick in the butt, and return to gratefulness and thankfulness. Sometimes that worked and sometimes it did not. I found that changing activities, visiting with people I love, doing something active, were all helpful in jogging the blues. Sometimes a nap or going to sleep for the night was the only thing that helped, and then waking up the next morning, I was again grateful to be alive and focused on being thankful for every minute I received. It sure felt better than moaning "poor me" and as much as I could, I continued to focus on this gratefulness for the entire sixteen weeks of chemo and beyond.

That first day of chemo treatment I came with a full entourage. My husband and two of my daughters were eager to accompany me and I was happy that they came along. Later in the morning, my family physician/friend dropped in for a visit. All came bearing gifts of food – homemade cookies, sandwiches, and a gorgeous fruit platter. It was a veritable party. I was a little worried that perhaps we were too rowdy, possibly disturbing some of the other patients in the large day treatment room who might have preferred quiet. Nobody complained, and many actually seemed to appreciate the distraction and the food that we passed around. The hospital I went to is a very welcoming one, and the staff certainly tried to make the chemo ordeal a more bearable one. To help pass the time there were massage therapists available, an art therapist, a woman who came in weekly to play the harp, and volunteers who brought rolling carts of food, along with good cheer, creating an atmosphere which was anything but grim. Every time I came in for treatment I made sure to book a massage, and gave myself over to the wonderful volunteers who did reflexology or shiatsu as the chemicals streamed into my body.

As a naturally garrulous person, I was eager to speak to women around me going through the same experiences I was. While not everybody in the room had breast cancer, there were several who were easily identifiable by their bald heads and the bright color of the drip flowing through their arms, and it was easy to strike up conversations. Friendships were formed, telephone numbers exchanged and informal support groups were created. Comparing notes on what we were going through, learning from the veterans, and cheering each other on, formed the basis of a unique bond forged by our common plight. To this day, I am in active contact with several of the woman I met while in chemo and my connection them has become very deep and strong. While outsiders were kind, caring and solicitous, the feeling prevailed that only somebody who has been there can really understand. Kvetching with fellow travelers along the cancer path was completely self-affirming and helpful in a way that only somebody who has been there and done that can understand. While many people find this kind of support in more formal, organized support groups, for me this informal network was just right.

Accompanying each chemo treatment, I received a big dose of steroids and some potent anti-nausea medication that nobody had actually spent time explaining to me. The anti-nausea medicine was easy to understand, but why the steroids? Apparently, they were there to help with the chemo side effects, but of course, they often have side effects of their own. I found that the "wired" feeling they gave me was unpleasant, but tolerable.

When my first treatment was finished, at about three o'clock in the afternoon, I was surprised to find that I felt a bit shaky and unsteady on my feet. I had figured that it was going to take a while to start having any reactions. My husband drove me home and I began to feel much worse. I got into bed for a short nap, and I woke up feeling terrible. I had never felt this bad in my life. Was it going to get worse? Was this as bad as it would get? What was next? This unnerving state made me extremely anxious and tense and I felt myself entering a downward spiral. Using guided imagery to calm myself down was somewhat helpful, but I still felt awful. Eating was not an option. I had no appetite and the idea of food was nauseating, even though I was not actually nauseous. I felt like I was jumping out of my skin and did not know what to do. I could not sleep. I could not focus enough to read or even watch a movie. I could not do much of anything. I found that while listening to my iPod I could drift in and out of consciousness and that helped me get through the really bad first few hours. That first night my Chinese medicine/acupuncturist was kind enough to come to my house and give me a treatment in bed. I had called her earlier and told her how bad I felt, so bad in fact that I could not move off the bed. After the acupuncture treatment, I felt an immediate improvement and that was very reassuring. This reminded me that the symptoms would eventually recede. I know that sounds obvious, but when you are in the midst of experiencing horrible new symptoms you are sure they will last forever. Everything was so new and frightening at that point. Anything that I could do to relax myself, and remind myself that I was still me, even though I did not feel like me, was good. I, similar to most people I know, like to feeling in control of situations, and chemo is a situation where one is clearly not in control. The way I adapted to my "new" life after the first treatment was by adjusting my expectations. Now that I had the experience of one treatment under my belt, I thought that I understood what to expect. I figured that allowing each treatment to be followed by a certain number of days "off" from my regular activities including work, housekeeping, food preparation, and family responsibilities, was a reasonable expectation. These were the days I would "kick back" and do nothing. To some degree, this was true, but in fact there were many ups and downs, and no two chemo treatments had the same effect on me.

Back to "kicking back" and doing "nothing." Doing nothing? It turns out that I am not very good at that. All my life I have been a really active person. Raising seven children while juggling a challenging career leaves virtually no down time. What little spare time I had I filled with exercise, reading and social activities with friends. I come from a strong tradition of doing, accomplishing, and moving. My parents idea of a day off was taking a car trip to some interesting destination, or visiting several museums. This "doing nothing" was entirely new to me. My immediate goal became passing the time until I would feel better and could pick up my regular activities. What could help me with this? I needed distractions to help me pass the time because, unfortunately, I have always been impatient with waiting. I hate long lines in the supermarket and have been known to leave a full cart if the wait is too long. I will drive great detours to avoid traffic jams. Now I found myself just sitting on the sofa, waiting, waiting, waiting for time to pass. Just waiting.

So how DID the time pass? I took my morning walk just about every day, thanks to my walking partner who matched her steps to mine. When I was slow, she just walked slowly by my side. If I was unsteady, I hung on to her. She was amenable to my walking at whatever time suited me. Early mornings were always best, but sometimes morning began at 6 and sometimes at 7. Fortunately, we had begun the walking regimen about two months before chemo began, so we had a good routine, and an excellent route, walking in the nearby rural community that gives us city folks a chance to breathe some fresh air and watch the unfolding of nature as the seasons change.

After my daily walk was done, I felt a sense of accomplishment, something that I had taken for granted but now realized how much I treasure. Since I had already accomplished something for the day, I could allow myself to let go a bit, and try my hand at the business of "doing nothing". Checking those emails I never had time for when I was a working girl, surfing the internet and watching TV are definitely good time wasters. As I write these words I realize that "time wasters" are words that belong to people in the workaday world. I had crossed that line. I was no longer one of them. I inhabited the world of the sick, the infirm, and the handicapped. Much as I didn't like to see myself in that way, the days after chemo were days when I needed to allow myself to be there, and I needed to reassure myself that I wasn't merely wasting time. I was recuperating! I was stopping that cancer short in its tracks and healing.

That feeling of my having crossed a line apparently bothered one of my friends almost more than it bothered me. She gave me a tongue lashing about using the word "sick." I was not to say that I was "sick." I could say, according to her, that I had a disease but I, Naomi Baum, was not sick. I was surprised by her   vehement reaction. On one level, I accepted it, and even believed it. I did not feel like a sick person. Yes, I was weak. Yes I felt terrible, and couldn't concentrate, or go to work or do much of anything. All true. But my soul didn't feel sick. At my core I didn't feel like a sick person. So I understood what she was saying and appreciated that she was saying this to make me feel stronger and better.

On the other hand, I found her criticism extremely offensive. I tried to tell myself that her words came from a good place, a place of caring and love, but I thought that it was a strange way to express that caring. I did want and need attention for being sick. I wanted people to be nice to me, to call me, to visit me. I deserved it. I WAS sick. What was this business about me not using the word sick? Was it her fears and anxieties coming to play? Why was she throwing them at me??

I found myself saying, "I have cancer," rather than "I am a cancer patient," as if that would keep that yucky old cancer external to me and outside of my core. The difference between saying "I have cancer" and "I am a cancer patient" may seem subtle but to me it felt that if you are a cancer patient that's all you are – it defines your whole self – whereas if you have cancer, it's just one aspect of yourself among the many. You have a whole self plus cancer.

However, if I am entirely truthful, and I try to be, I most certainly was a cancer patient as well, and the cancer was inside of me. And yes, I was sick. I hoped to get over it and move on. I most definitely did not think that was all I was, although there were days when that was all I was. There was a certain comfort in giving myself over to where I was at the moment. From all my readings and from my practice of mindfulness, I knew that staying alertly in the present brings a certain amount of peace and steadiness. Appreciating where I was in the moment and not glossing over it, even if that moment was both uncomfortable and difficult, was healing for me.

The fact that I had stepped over the line from the world of healthy, carefree, unknowing people into the netherworlds of cancer became apparent to all when my hair and eyebrows fell out. I was a marked woman. I could try to cover up my balding head, but what could I do to replace eyelashes?? The interesting thing is that I did not actually notice when they fell out (or the rest of my body hair, and I mean ALL my body hair). It just kind of happened, and I only noticed after it was gone. The hair on my head was a different story. There I tracked the steady progress of my hair loss over the course of about a week between my second and third chemo treatment. Because my hair was so short it was a lot less dramatic than it might have been, and I merely found my pillow covered with whiskers of hair for a couple of days. Because it was entirely even, I decided to shave my scalp entirely, to get a nice smooth effect, and once I did that, I was no longer preoccupied with the reminder of hairs falling out. Many women tell me that their scalp itches and is painful when their hair falls out. I did not experience any of that, perhaps because my hair was so short.

Initially I was a bit embarrassed about my bald head, and it definitely took some getting used to. I would wake up in the morning and look at myself in the mirror and say, "who is that?" Did you ever wonder what you would look like without hair? Well it turns out that I had a nice scalp, rather round and well formed. It was a bald head to be proud of! After finding the wig I had bought for this occasion intolerable, I began covering my balding head with stylish scarves and hats. It was fun for a while, but at some point became tedious. By this point, I was much more used to the idea of me being bald and actually was finding it interesting and fun. I know that sounds weird, but that is the truth. I ventured out bald and found that I loved it. It was certainly a conversation piece, and I felt good. I got loads of compliments (Were people just being nice? Who cared?). I have always liked being a little different from the crowd, and this was definitely one way to go about it.

Chemo lasted for sixteen long weeks. I sent e-mail updates regularly during this time, and I will let my letters speak for me during this intense period of my healing journey.

Update # 11 – September 1

Hi all,

Another update from the trenches....

I am sitting in an arm chair in the day treatment oncology center on the seventh floor at Sha'arei Zedek, waiting....

That's the story here – a lot of patience.

The way it works is that we get here around 8, take a number, wait for a blood test, take the blood sample down to the lab, and then wait to make sure my blood counts are ok. If they are (and hopefully they are), they order up the meds.

There are all sorts of interesting things to keep one busy: art therapy, massage, spiritual care, and visits from friends and family. Today Shlomzi drove me here, Shoshi is coming in the middle and Mike is picking me up, so I am well cared for and well entertained. As you see by my writing this e-mail, there are computers here to also help pass the time. Actually the most interesting thing for me (as always) is the people – and their interesting stories. That IS why I became a psychologist, and one of these days I may start writing down some of the stories I've heard.

The last two weeks passed relatively well. The first few days after the chemo were a bit rocky, up and down, with very strange and weird feelings, rather hard to describe. Maybe by the second time I will be able to describe them better. I schlepped around for the better part of a week, but in that time I did manage to go to the movies, to an artist fair, out to dinner a few times. I worked for a few hours a day the first week post-chemo, and then full days the second week, and I even managed to take a two-day vacation with Shlomzi. We decided to go to Mizpe Ramon to escape the crowds in the north (the shooting in the south did make for a quiet time), and decided that because Mizpe is at a very high elevation the weather would be good, and it was. We stayed at the Pundak Ramon, a very nice hotel with a pool and excellent food. Having a pool so accessible encouraged me to go swimming for the first time in months, and I found it both invigorating and great for my arm post-surgery. Since then I have rejoined the local pool, and gone swimming twice, including early this morning before heading out for chemo. Shlomzi and I decided to explore the more remote places around the crater, and we visited several farms, including one that had goats and made wonderful cheese, a winery, and an outpost on the Egyptian border where we met an artist who makes beautiful jewelry (we bought some). We even had a massage. The scenery was great, the company outstanding, and we had a wonderful time. By Friday, ten days post chemo, I was back to myself (relief, relief) and we went to the gym and the movies. One of the interesting things I have noticed over the past week is how I feel like I have to push everything in before the next round of chemo. That includes: work, house, kids, family, friends, errands, etc, etc. So the last few days have been very busy – but good - and now I will have the enforced rest that comes with the chemo. Last time round I found that I wasn't much good for anything for a few days, and visits were a welcome distraction. So if you are around the neighborhood, give a call, and see if I am up for it – or just come by. If I am not friendly, or need to sleep – I will tell you, don't worry. That is one of the things about cancer – it allows you to "tell it like it is" and people accept it.

So wish me luck. Hopefully my blood counts are good, and I will get the chemo today, and be 25% finished with this interesting journey. Once again, thank God I live in an age and country where this cutting edge treatment is available to me, thank God for my wonderful medical team, thank God for my wonderful family and friends.

Update # 12 -September 14

Hi all,

It's been quite a ride these last two weeks.

I had chemo two weeks ago today (Thurs), and was hobbling along, and had just ended a pleasant, quiet Shabbat when we got the sad news that Mike's father passed away on Friday night. The next week was a very intense week – funeral on Sunday, Shiva (the Jewish ritual mourning period of seven days) in Ra'anana from Sunday to Tuesday with Mike's sister and mom, and then at home with Mike's Aunt Norma, till late Friday afternoon. Thank God I had the strength and stamina to participate in all of it. I bless my father-in-law that he chose this week, because I knew it was good for me to have distractions and visitors the week after chemo – and in fact there were lots of those that week. It was also incredible to hear Mike talk about his dad, encompassing his entire life, recapturing the vital and principled man that he was, a man of quiet warmth, deep thoughts, and strong convictions.

And then, after a very busy Shabbat (Saturday, the Jewish day of rest) with Chana and company (Jason and 4 kids), it was back to a regular week filled mostly with work, and "catch up" on the rest of my life. So far – after two rounds of chemo – it seems that I am reasonably knocked out for a week, staying close to home with the option of lying down every couple of hours for a short rest, and in between doing a bit of work, staying on top of e-mails, visiting, etc. I am doing a fair amount of guided imagery which I am finding very helpful, and have returned to swimming and exercise – not in the immediate aftermath of chemo, but picking up a few days later. The swimming has been just wonderful to rehabilitate my arm after surgery, and my friend Noga has been very faithful about taking me for walks every morning.

Mike and I are taking advantage of a few more days "off" to go up to Kibbutz Lavi, to participate in the wedding of our good friends' son, with a mini-vacation thrown in for good measure. We continue to enjoy our blessings, and take nothing (or not much) for granted.

Shabbat shalom – be well dear friends and family,

Naomi

Update #13-September 25

Dear Family and Friends,

This year instead of the traditional "Baum Rosh Hashana letter" an update and best wishes for a shana tova, a happy new year, will have to suffice. In the plethora of e-cards and e-wishes for a sweet year, I hope this letter will still find its way to you with all of my heartfelt wishes for a year filled with blessings to each and every one of you and your families. It is at times like this that the rather mundane wishes for health and peace take on so much more meaning. So yes – I bless each and every one of you with good health, with peace within and peace without – for each one of you individually, and to all of us.

So what have we? I am moving along on this road that seems to be stretching on into the distance at this point. It kind of reminds me of "sophomore slump". The beginning seems like a long time ago, the end of treatment is still not in sight, and yet if I focus on each day and each moment. For the most part, life is good, full, interesting, and yes...even fun. I continue to be amazed by my immediate family and friends, near and far – how much your support is both so meaningful and helpful. I am overwhelmed by requests to accompany me to chemo (it's not so great...it just sounds like a lot of fun), offers for food and all kinds of other help. One of the lessons I am learning is how to ask for help, and how to say no thank you. Two sides of the coin that are sometimes difficult to navigate.

So the last week has again been up-and-down after the third round of chemo. It seems to have taken a little longer to "right" myself, but thankfully I have only one more dose of the AC, next Monday after Rosh Hashana, and then after that we start on the T (Taxol) which is supposed to be easier to bear for most folks. I have found that what helps me most on the more difficult days is distraction, and so I have thrown myself into that. I go to a wonderful class in Talmud in the nearby women's seminary, and I was able to attend the day after chemo for most of the morning, leaving a recorder to tape the part I missed. The following days I cajoled family members (Shoshi, Mike, Shlomzi) to take me out – checking out the various eateries around here, fig picking, and shopping. We stayed local so that I could crash at a moment's notice, which I find I need to do every couple of hours in the days immediately after chemo. What the distractions do is remind me that there is a lot more to me than just the big C, and I actually successfully forget about myself for hours at a time, which is a big relief. You have no idea how wearing it is to constantly be checking in with myself as to "how are you?" And speaking of "how are you?" I keep wondering how honest I need to be? Is there any advantage to saying "lousy"? Perhaps I should just say "ok" or "fine". Being a religious Jew has its advantages here,

because i have been finding that the response "baruch haShem" (thank God) is a good answer no matter how I feel. And it helps remind me to be grateful for being alive.

At this time of year when we all do an accounting of the year past and think about the year to come, we are truly thankful (and here I include Mike because I know he is with me on this) for our blessings. We had three grandchildren born this year, two of our kids finished the army, two of them finished their Bachelor's degrees, all of our grown children are working in meaningful jobs and raising beautiful families, and the younger ones are moving along and developing. That was the annual update! We hope that the year to come will bring to all of us, and that includes you, a year of continued blessings.

Much love,

Naomi

So routine takes over. Even during chemo. There is a natural rhythm, and even a sense of what to expect that develops after awhile. You know how many days since your last chemo. You know how many days until your next scheduled chemo. You know that you will feel bad for a certain number of days. The feeling bad part is actually the part that feels out of control. You don't know precisely how many days; you don't know exactly which side effects will kick in this time, or how your body will react. I found it surprising how eager I was to establish a baseline, to recapture a sense of control even with the side effects. I would say, "Last time I felt lousy for eight days, so I expect it will be the same this time." That gave me a perceived sense of control, and lasted until I got to the ninth day, at which point I felt even worse because I wasn't feeling better already, as planned.

I also developed a pattern related to various complementary medicine treatments I was doing:

- Acupuncture
- Shiatsu
- Lymphatic massage
- Regular massage
- Guided imagery

Cancer care really IS a full time job. Establishing this schedule gave me a sense of routine and routine naturally brings along with it a feeling of safety. I knew where I was going and what I was doing next, at least insofar as treatments were concerned.   But what really lay in wait for me around the corner?? Who knew? In a life that at its very core felt out of control, I was clutching at any semblance of control that I could. And if I might add, in a healthy way.

Update #14 – October 12

Dear friends and family,

It is the eve of Sukkot (the Jewish Festival of Booths) and the last of the cooking is done. It seems to me that it is a time for another update from down home on the ranch. Actually, it is good to be home. After spending the last three days vacationing away from home, it is always nice to come back, and I am always happy to notice that I am happy coming home. We were fortunate to be able to squeeze in a three-day vacation up in Kibbutz Lavi Guesthouse with our entire immediate family (sans Shuey, who is living it up in Dar es Salaam, Tanzania – check out the blog if you haven't already: www.naomibaum.wordpress.com). We didn't over-plan the vacation, not knowing exactly how I would feel, so in terms of programming it was rather low key, but that meant that there was plenty of time to hang out, and just be with each other, which in fact was the purpose of the whole adventure. Kibbutz Lavi provided a wonderful backdrop.   Nice rooms, grass, pool, good food, playground, and the kids provided the entertainment. The weather was quite hot, so we took advantage of water – we went to the beach on Sunday, the pool on Monday, and yesterday concluded the vacation at a natural swimming hole called Ein Nun. There was even a hike for the hikers, who climbed up a big mountain (I wasn't there, so couldn't tell you the name of the mountain)   while   we   non-hikers enjoyed making perfumed soap, and walking around Bet Lehem Haglilit, one of the original Templar settlements.

Our vacation was preceded by Rosh Hashana and Yom Kippur. Rosh Hashana is by now a distant memory. Mostly what I remember is that it was long, many meals, too much food, and very good company. Mike initiated a discussion at the table on Friday night (meal number 5) about what each one of us plans to take on themselves for the year to come. What surprised me most was how each person at the table (and we were around 14) participated, and shared. For me it was a difficult question – mainly, because i didn't want to cry. I tend to cry quite easily these days and, while I have gotten more or less used to the tears, it still sometimes embarrasses me in front of larger groups. So I was happy that I had a bit of time to mull over it. And then I waffled, saying only part of what I really wanted to. So I have been thinking about this question ever since and here is my chance. This is what I want to take on this year:

I want to take on a complete healing. I want to lick this damn cancer so hard that it doesn't even think about coming back. So this year I am taking on healing and health. That is in addition to my very public commitment (and this I did say at the table) to write a book. The question then is: a book about what? I am still searching for the answer to that. I have three different starts, and that is what they are – starts. Fits and starts. So we will see, and wonder whether public commitments such as these actually do make a difference.

And then on to treatment number four, the Monday after Rosh Hashana, and after that, Yom Kippur. Treatment number four was about the same as the other three, except that the side effects do seem to become more pronounced, and last longer, despite my valiant efforts to up the acupuncture, add shiatsu, and do whatever I can on the complementary medicine side of things. I am hopeful that the next four treatments (in which Taxol replaces the Doxorubicin and Cyclophosphamide will be kinder to me. I am so hopeful in fact, that Shlomzi and I have ordered tickets for a concert on Monday night (the day of my next treatment). Actually, the way I figure it is that the concert will be sold out, and worst comes to worst, Shlomzi will be able to sell my ticket, or find a friend to go with.

Which brings us up to the present. The sukkah (A temporary hut constructed for the holiday week, in which all meals are eaten) is ready, the food is cooked and the company is on their way. We are looking forward to a holiday of "simcha" – happiness and joy. The harvest is in , we are ready for the winter, and we are moving out to our sukkah, our temporary booth, to look up to the heavens and remind ourselves that we are all in God's hands.

Wishing you all a joyful holiday,

With love,

Naomi

Update #15 – November 8

Dear Friends and Family,

It has been quite a while since I have written- at least a month or so, and again I can tell because I have been getting many calls and e-mails. So in considering why I haven't written, I think the answer is that I have entered a certain routine. The cancer is old news by now. Chemo is also "been there, done that", and life goes on. But for those of you that I communicate with less regularly, a short update is nevertheless in order.

I have completed six of the eight planned treatments. I am now receiving Taxol, which has different side effects than the first four treatments. The side effects of Taxol are so far easier for me to handle and shorter in duration, which makes for a better lifestyle. One of the things I find so interesting about chemo, though, is that you never quite know what to expect, or when. So last week I had chemo on Monday, was feeling very well on Tuesday, well into Wednesday morning and then, all of a sudden I felt BAD, in the middle of the day. After some painkillers and a big nap, I pulled myself together enough to go to the wedding of children of dear friends, and was so happy to be able to participate, but I cancelled plans for Thursday and laid low most of the day, until Mike came home to entertain me. By the weekend I was more or less back to myself, and here I am sitting in a restaurant waiting for my daughters and daughters-in-law to join me for dinner. The excuse: a coupon for a sushi restaurant. We'll grab at any excuse these days to celebrate.

In considering what to share with you in this update, I was thinking of all the benefits of cancer. Why was I thinking about this? I was just realizing that I am thankfully nearing the end of chemo, and while there is still a ways to go (more surgery and a course of radiation), the end of chemo will be a milestone, and feels like significant progress.

So what are the benefits of cancer? Here is my partial, and growing, list:

1. People are very nice to you (by people I mean, starting with family, neighbors, friends, and ending with the cop who stopped me the other day, and when she saw how bald I was, let me go!)

2. I push myself less hard and spoil myself more. In short, I am nicer to myself.

3. I do only the things I want to (for the most part) e.g. if there's a work meeting I'd rather not attend – I pass on it.

4. I get lots of massages (many at reduced prices).

5. I think daily about my purpose in life. I don't know if the net result is living a more "considered life" but I think there may be some potential here.

6. I am regularly grateful for all that I have, and all that God has given me.

7. I work less and take more time for other parts of my life - learning, exercise, family.

So that's the beginning of the growing list. Feel free to add your suggestions – I am sure there are more.

Thanks again for all your interest, love, prayers and support – it all helps. I know it.

Love,

Naomi

December 12, 2011

Update # 16 - December 1

Hi all,

As things have reached a certain equilibrium, and life has taken on a semblance of normal routine, I have had, thank God less news to report on, and haven't written in a while. My last chemo, a somewhat non-event in the life of the seventh floor Day Oncology Unit, was a mega-event in my book, and my vibes must have reached all my kids, because many of them made an effort to be there and celebrate with me. The thing is, the medicine that I have been receiving these last two months, Taxol, is given with several other medications to reduce the chance for allergic reaction (which thankfully I never had). Those medications made me extremely sleepy and sent me off to the auxiliary rooms that have beds, away from the "big room" where all the action is. I tried to warn my kids that it would be relatively boring. The harpist, the food wagons and all the other entertainment that rolls in and out of the seventh floor to help the patients pass their time more pleasantly, more or less skip over the auxiliary rooms. No matter. The kids showed up and partied as I slept on. I woke up for a slice of pizza they ordered (a new twist on the term "hospital delivery"), and for the final half hour of chemo. When the dedicated nurse (and they are a wonderful, dedicated bunch – I am still trying to figure out how to say a proper thank you to them. Ideas?) pulled out my final IV, we all broke out into song, and sang a medley of our favorite songs for about twenty minutes. The medley started with my granddaughter's favorite song that had become a theme song for me this year, thanking God for all the goodness He has heaped on me. Patients and staff stuck their heads in to see what the commotion was about and left smiling.

So, that was it for chemo.

But let me paint the background picture to that day. After
several months of chemo I finally finessed the system, and rather than getting to the hospital early to do blood tests and then wait and wait and wait until the test results were okayed, the medicine ordered, and delivered, I finally figured out that the day before chemo I could do a finger stick blood test at the local clinic two blocks from my house, and save several hours of waiting on the day of chemo. After getting the lab results back, faxing them over to the hospital and getting them okayed, you need to call in on the morning of chemo to tell the nurses you intend to show up (was that a choice??) and then show up about 11 AM. I used the time to good advantage, to attend a yoga class that I began going to several weeks ago. So picture that: yoga from 7:30-10:30, and then a quick drive over to the hospital for chemo. Quite the contrast, no?

I actually spent not a small amount of time considering how I wanted to celebrate the end of chemo. Clearly it is but one step along the path, and I am not finished yet (is one ever "finished"?) but to my mind any reason to stop, give thanks, be grateful, and celebrate, is reason enough to do just that. I spent a lot of time imagining all sorts of celebrations, but have decided that this one would be fairly low key, and modest. We had a family dinner the other night with the kids and that was lovely, and special. I will "bench gomel" this Shabbat or next – meaning, that I will say a special blessing in synagogue on Sabbath thanking God for all the good He has given me. And I mean that! And of course, Mike and I are going on vacation. I will save the bigger celebration for a later date.

I have lots more to say- but this is getting very long- so i will save more for the next letter, which may come quicker than the last. So let me just take this opportunity to wish you all a happy Hanukah and Shabbat shalom.Much love – and thanks for your concern, interest, prayers, love, etc, etc.

Naomi

And that about sums it up for chemo.

TIPS FOR GETTING THROUGH CHEMO:

1. Find areas in life where you feel in control and make the most of them.

2. Explore complementary medicine to help with side effects.

3. Line up friends and family for the help you think you might need.

4. Learn to ask for help.

5. Learn to set limits and tell people if/when you need to rest, or just want some time alone.

6. Make time for vacation as the chemo allows. Chemo is now your day job, and occasionally you need a vacation from that, too.

7. Involve your kids in your treatment as much as you feel comfortable.

8. Find five things to be grateful for EVERY SINGLE DAY. Write them down. If you are having trouble getting to five, start with two and build up from there. It doesn't matter how small or trivial the item is. Write it down.

[10]

Decision Making

Update #17- December 8

I will be having surgery a week from Monday (Dec 19):   *a re-lumpectomy, which means a relatively small surgery, to take out more breast tissue, because the margins the first time round were too close. For those of you for whom this makes no sense: tumors are taken out with some tissue surrounding the tumor. The idea is to have at least some healthy, non-cancerous tissue all the way around. In my first surgery one side of the tumor was too close to the margin, so they will go back in to "clean out" and hopefully come out with clean margins. I debated long and hard between a re-lumpectomy and a mastectomy, which was an option, and opted for the smaller surgery at this time. This does not rule out having a mastectomy somewhere down the road but at this point in time, with recommendations both from my surgeon and oncologist. I am comfortable with the smaller surgery, and don't – at least at this point in time – have to deal with the more difficult sequelae of losing a breast.*

I t sounds like the decision was a simple one. It wasn't. One of the great challenges of having cancer at this point in man's evolution is the need to make many medical decisions. Fifty or one hundred years ago, when a lot less was known, there were far fewer choices to be made. Along with gratefulness for all the latest medical breakthroughs, diagnostic and imaging techniques, and new treatment protocols, comes the need to make decisions. Additionally, since patients have become more proactive in their care, doctors have learned that it is important to involve the patient in the decision making process.

Once again I was at a point in my illness where decisions had to be made. Once again I debated long and hard, this time between a re-lumpectomy and a mastectomy. Earlier the debate had been between a lumpectomy and a mastectomy. At the end of the day, I once again opted for the smaller surgery. Compared to my earlier decision, this decision was a soul searching, more difficult decision to make.

Let me backtrack. My initial decision to place the bulk of my care in the hands of two dedicated physicians, my surgeon and oncologist, was made without a lot of angst. There was virtually no discussion about treatment protocols and types of chemo, and I felt comfortable with that, as I was being treated with the standard breast cancer treatment, about which everyone was in agreement. My original surgery was a lumpectomy. I consulted with two surgeons before the lumpectomy and they both thought that this was a good choice in my situation. We discussed the option of mastectomy but both surgeons felt that it was not necessary and thus, while I did have to make the final decision, it was not such a difficult one for me to make. With both surgeons recommending lumpectomy, I breathed a sigh of relief and signed on.

However, when the pathology results came back from the initial surgery, they showed that the margins of the tumor that was
removed were not clean. In other words, there was not enough healthy, cancer-free tissue surrounding the tumor to assure both the surgeon and me that all the cancer had been removed. It was clear that I would need to have further surgery and the only question was how extensive the surgery should be. Mastectomy or lumpectomy? Lumpectomy or mastectomy?

My surgeon weighed in on the side of lumpectomy, my oncologist was equivocal and the second opinion surgeon thought I should do a mastectomy this time round. Now I was in a pickle. What was I to do? How does one decide something like this? Each one of the physicians I consulted with concluded his consultation session by saying that it was a very personal decision, and one that I would have to make alone. Couldn't they decide for me?? Why did I have to make the decision? Alone? For a while there I was ready to go back to the days of the authoritarian physician who sits on a seat close to God and makes all the decisions for you.

In trying to deconstruct this decision, I tried to unravel the web that I seemed to be caught in. What was going on? First and
foremost there was my very strong will to live. I would do anything that would ensure me a longer, disease free life. Initially I thought that a mastectomy would give me that peace of mind, and insurance against a recurrence. I was so excited about the idea that I could be cancer-free forever and never worry again, that for a short while I even entertained the notion of doing a bilateral mastectomy in order to assure myself of a long and disease free life.

However, the more I delved into the matter and read about it, the less clear it became, and there were absolutely no guarantees
attached to performing a mastectomy. Did you know that women who have mastectomies still have a risk of getting breast cancer on the side that was removed? I was told by my physician that there is always a chance that not all the cancer cells were removed from the remaining tissue. So, if I were to have a mastectomy, I would still need to undergo radiation. Regardless of my decision, I would also still need regular monitoring with breast exams, ultrasound and possibly mammography and MRI. My risk of reoccurrence would drop by a few percentage points, but nobody could guarantee me a clean bill of health, so the net gain would not be as great as I had hoped.

As the waters were muddying and things were becoming a lot less clear, my self -image took center stage. What is self-image made of? I imagine it to be layers and layers of thoughts, feelings, pictures and perceptions that probably have their roots way back in childhood. One of the more prominent features right now was my femininity; what I think about my breasts, how important were they to me? How would I feel without them? I did not have a clue as to how to go about answering these questions. I just knew my breasts were there. I had not given them all that much thought probably since I was a teenager, or maybe when I was a breastfeeding young mother. I knew that deep down I really do care about how I look even though I spend minimal time on self-grooming, makeup, and fussing about my looks. I pride myself on being a take-it-or-leave-it kind of gal. What you see is what you get, and what you get is the REAL me, without much artifice. But I'm not oblivious to my appearance. So where were these circular thoughts leading me? How was I ever going to make a decision?

Eventually, the winning point as far as I was concerned was made by my surgeon, who told me that I would be a lot more uncomfortable with the mastectomy as compared to the lumpectomy. In his words, my quality of life post-surgery would be significantly better with a lumpectomy, and that had to do with the fact that I wear a D cup. He explained that because I am so "big" (I had never considered myself big, just nicely endowed), I would feel unbalanced by having one breast removed and might experience significant discomfort. When I brought up the notion of bilateral mastectomy, he said there was absolutely no indication to remove the healthy breast, and he would not consider it at this time. It was clear that if I was going to go forward with the notion of a bilateral mastectomy I would have to change surgeons.

When discussing this issue with my oncologist, I finally understood that his main concern was not a recurrence of breast cancer in the same breast or the other breast (for which I do have a higher risk, now that I "got" it once). The big worry was, and continues to be, metastases in various parts of my body, because I had seven infected lymph nodes. Mastectomy was not going to solve that worry in any way, shape or form. Opening my eyes to this real state of affairs, presented to me in no uncertain terms, was both unsettling and scary. While I was busy worrying about lumpectomy or mastectomy, the real question was, were there metastases lurking in my body? Why hadn't I thought about that before? Denial? Fear?

When the oncologist spoke to me so forthrightly, and it became clear to me that essentially my ruminations were a side issue, I opted for a re-lumpectomy. Ultimately, I decided that since I did not know what life had in store for me, I would rather live what life is granted to me as best I can. For me that meant living with as little surgical intervention as possible.   This whole process of decision-making took place over the course of approximately two months, while I was going through chemo, because the surgery was to take place approximately three weeks after I completed chemo.   During this time, aside from consulting physicians, I talked my husband's ear off, drew up lists of pros and cons, journaled, talked to women who had been through mastectomies, and gingerly foraged on the internet.   The women I spoke to were very emphatic in their feelings that what they had done had been the right thing for them.   Most were careful not to impose their decisions on me, but I did get the feeling that no matter what one decides, it is important to live well with that decision.

In addition to all of these avenues that I explored in an effort to reach a decision, I tried to focus inward.   By sitting quietly and waiting for an inner voice to make itself known I thought I might be able to figure out what was right for me.   After all, everybody agreed that this was a very personal decision that only I could make.   While I must confess I did not have one moment of revelation, the more I sat with it, the more comfortable I felt with the decision to have the lumpectomy.   I figured that, in the worst-case scenario, I could always do a mastectomy later on down the road.   At least for now I would opt for the more minimal surgery that would require very little in terms of recuperation and rehabilitation.   The re-lumpectomy involved reopening the original scar, scooping out some more tissue and sending it to a pathology lab for testing. Much to my delight and surprise the surgery this time round was a piece of cake, and seemed much easier than the first surgery.   For starters, there was no drain, no underarm pain, and the healing was quick. Surprisingly, I was not as preoccupied with the pathology results as I had been the first time round. I did not count the days waiting to hear from the doctor. Was this denial? If so, it wasn't such a bad thing. I was actually surprised that my surgeon seemed a lot less laid back about the pathology results than I was. On my post-surgical follow-up visit he profusely apologized for not having the results, which I hadn't expected to begin with, and then told me to call him in two or three days to see if the results had arrived. Before I even had a chance to call him I received a call from his surgical nurse in the OR. She told me that the surgeon was in the middle of surgery, but had a big smile on his face because he had just gotten some good news. All the tissue he had taken out was cancer free! Rather than jumping for joy, I accepted the results very matter-of-factly and returned to my yoga class that had been interrupted. Thinking over my response later in the day, in contrast to the reaction of the surgeon and his nurse, I began to worry that this might be the "flat affect" or "emotional detachment" that psychologists talk about when they write about traumatized individuals. Was I in fact emotionally detached? Was the experience I was going through so difficult and stressful, that the only way for me to deal with it was to become emotionally numb? I didn't think so, but I wasn't sure, and thought that it was worth contemplating and tracking. Reflecting on my lack of response from the perspective of time, I think that once I had made my decision, I was determined not to look back. I knew that if the results the second time round were not "clean", there was a good likelihood for mastectomy. I had been told that the chances for this were slim, but they did exist. Fortunately, I was able to focus on the upside of having "only" a re-lumpectomy, and I was blessed with very little second-guessing and rumination after I made my decision. Clearly, not everyone is so lucky. The factors that went in to my decision – comfort, quality of life, lack of real medical gain to be had from full mastectomy, were unique to me, and each women facing this decision will have factors unique to her and her disease. The fact that there is no one RIGHT decision cannot be said strongly enough and is not to be trivialized. This is thorny territory that each woman must explore herself. No matter how much support you may have, no matter how many advisors you may be surrounded with, the bottom line is that you are alone with yourself as you make this decision. Often the pros and cons can be very confusing, and the pressures mount as the decision becomes urgent. While this chapter has dealt with breast cancer and the decisions I had to make, the tips below relate to all types of cancers, and decisions that may have to do with various kinds of treatments from chemo protocols, to surgery, to follow-up. One thing to keep in mind is that decisions are always difficult, but in the end they have to be made. Below are some suggestions that may aid you in your decision making process.

TIPS FOR MAKING MEDICAL DECISIONS:

1. Write out all your questions, no matter how trivial.

2. Talk to your physicians again and again. Don't be afraid of them and don't be afraid to ask them anything. This is their job. Find out how they prefer that you contact them – whether by e-mail, cell phone, or office phone line - but do not hesitate to "bother" them. I am repeating this because so often we think we are a bother, when in fact the need to question and discuss is very legitimate, and addressing your concerns is part of your physician's job.

3. When things get confusing, take out a pencil and pad of paper and make a list of pros and cons. Revisit this list over a few days.

4. Talk to people who have your type of cancer and have experienced your various options. I spoke to women who had had mastectomies and lumpectomies. Most were very open and willing to talk about their experiences.

5. When you finish talking to everybody, sit with yourself in a quiet place and see what comes up for you. Do you have an inner preference for one of the options? If nothing comes up, wait, and try again.

6. Sit with your decision for a while. Even though time may be pressing, try not to make a hasty decision. The bottom line is that your decision has to feel right to you.

7. Once you have made your decision, try not to look back. While this may be easier said than done, second guessing can be very insidious. Each time you catch yourself thinking "what if" or "perhaps I should have", try to pull yourself back to the present, and ground yourself by taking a deep breath and finding something to be grateful for right now. Focus on all the reasons that support the decision you did make. Do NOT focus on the down side of your decision.

[11]

Work

This past week was a relatively peaceful one on the home front. I went to work several days – and here is the place to acknowledge how wonderful and supportive my boss and co-workers have been to me, right from the start. It is a wonderful environment to work in, and an even more wonderful environment to get sick in! Each and every person there has taken an interest in my wellbeing and shared smiles, hugs and words of encouragement, while picking up the inevitable slack in my work. During this period of chemo, I hope to continue part-time, combining work from home with days in the office, depending on how I feel. Of course even though this is the plan, I know that we will all need to be very flexible, as we are just at the beginning and learning every day.

I am a psychologist and I work in a non-profit trauma center, the Israel Center for the Treatment of Psychotrauma, in Jerusalem. I have worked at the Center for over ten years and am one of the senior professionals on staff. Over the years I have been cognizant of the fact that I am blessed in having a wonderful work environment, interesting work, supportive colleagues and a very understanding and flexible boss. There could not be a better recipe for helping someone with cancer than to work in an environment like this. When I was diagnosed, I immediately shared the news with my boss and closest colleagues and was given the clear message that they would support me and help me out in whatever way they could.

I spent the first month post-diagnosis in a relative daze. Although, I continued to drive to work every day and sit at my desk for a full work day, in fact, much of my efforts were spent squeezing in doctor appointments, diagnostic tests and trying to digest what was happening to me. As my productivity plummeted, and my ability to complete tasks diminished, my colleagues quietly picked up the pieces where I left off. After my initial diagnosis the pace of medical activity picked up and as I began to contemplate surgery and the inevitable treatment that would follow, it was clear to me that I would need to both take some time off and rearrange my schedule. I was not sure how to go about doing this. I was receiving all kinds of advice, both from people who had been through this and others who thought they knew what was good for me. There were those who said how important it was to keep working, while others suggested taking a leave of absence. What to do?

Once again, I needed to remind myself that each individual is unique, and what works for one person may be an absolute disaster for another. This concept has been a recurring theme in this book because I found it to be one of the most important lessons of my cancer journey. In some ways, I thought, it would be easier if there was a tried-and-true prescription to follow that would work for all of us. But clearly there isn't one road and so figuring out whether to work, how much to work, and when to work, were all open questions that I was going to have to deal with in my own way.

Interestingly, many people are eager to offer opinions on this matter. The most common piece of advice, and one that I heard a lot, is that work is good for you and will help you take your mind off things. This may be true for some, but not for others, and I would certainly hesitate to offer this up unequivocally as a "truth." It is important for each one of us to find out what works for US as individuals. Some questions to ask ourselves that may help us find the road include: How are you feeling physically? How is the treatment affecting you? Are you physically able to get to work? Do you think it would be good for you? In addition, financial considerations can be critical and may drive your decision. Do you have paid sick leave? Do you have disability insurance? Is it enough to cover your expenses? What about job security? If you take off a long period of time will you have a job to come back to?

While cancer is certainly not something one chooses, silver linings occasionally make themselves known, and not infrequently in the field of work. This may be a serendipitous time to look at how much you really like your job. You can ask yourself whether you enjoy going to work. Do you enjoy the people at work? Is this the job that you want to come back to? During my year of treatment I met a woman who told me how cancer had liberated her from a job that she was chained to and a boss whom she had despised for over twenty years. She was practically singing the praises of cancer, saying that cancer was the best thing that ever happened to her. This may be a bit extreme, but since your life has taken a sharp turn anyway, you might want to take a few moments to consider where you are professionally, and if this is where you would like to be. Having said that, I do not think this is necessarily the time to make a big job move or take on a new project, but it certainly can be a time for adjustments, tuning up, and change. Alternatively, this may simply be the time to note that your job is an issue you want to revisit at a later date.

One friend of mine stopped working entirely when she got cancer, and dedicated herself to healing and just hanging out. Another friend did not miss a day of work, except for the one day every other week when she had chemo. She scheduled her chemo right before the weekend on the same day that I had chemo, giving her two days to recuperate, and she was back at her desk at the beginning of the work week, without missing a beat. This was particularly hard for me to stomach because while she was returning to work, I was just beginning my deep descent into feeling lousy. While she was at her desk feeling "a little tired", I was splayed out on the sofa in the prone position, groaning. All I could do was repeat the refrain, "People are different."

I tried very hard to listen inward, and to see if I could figure out what direction I wanted to take where work was concerned. After surgery, I decided to take three weeks off to recuperate, even though the surgeon said I could go back to work after only two weeks. After those initial two weeks, I found that I was still tired and not back to myself, and I felt that an extra week at home would do me good. Unlike my former pre-cancer self who never took a sick day, and would show up at work sniffling and coughing, I was listening to what my body needed and trying to take care of it. When it was clear that I would need chemo, I decided, with the support of my boss, not to make any hard-and-fast decisions but to play it by ear and see how things developed. At that early stage I had no idea how my body would react to the chemo, and how I would feel. The pattern that established itself fairly soon was that the first two days after chemo I felt pretty good, probably because I was still taking large doses of steroids, but by the third day I usually crashed and then stayed pretty low for about a week. During that week, I could answer e-mails and field urgent phone calls from work, but I couldn't imagine going in to the office daily and continuing work as usual. By the second week after chemo I was usually able to drag myself in to the office for several hours a day. By the time I was back to feeling really well it was only three or four days before my next treatment! Luckily for me, my staff was incredibly flexible and worked around my sporadic schedule.

The big benefit of going into the office and getting back to work was feeling normal for even just a little while. What work gave me was an escape from the world of cancer and illness, and entry into the world of health and productivity. For the few hours that I sat at my office desk and interacted with colleagues, I could pretend that my life that had not turned upside down, and was actually normal, just "business as usual." My colleagues played along with my charade and aside from a kind "how are you?" at the beginning of each day, and comments on my hair (or lack thereof), they allowed me to focus on work. It felt like a warm and welcome refuge.

My work at the Trauma Center has evolved over the years. I see very few clients, and at the time that I was diagnosed I had one active client. I found that I was not able to remain focused and present to the client's needs and quickly terminated treatment and referred the client to another therapist. Fortunately, the bulk of my work at the Trauma Center is more administrative in nature. I develop programs, write grants and reports, search for funding, and supervise staff members and teams who are actively working in the field. While the subject matter is often "traumatic" I am a few steps removed from the actual trauma most of the time. During my year of healing from cancer, my staff protected me and I was not directly involved in any interventions. I did not need more exposure to trauma in my life than I already had.

As trauma professionals, we are very cognizant of the impact of exposure to trauma on ourselves. Self-care, making sure to protect and support one's self is key to long term survival in the trauma field.

After completing chemo, I once again took off a block of time for my second surgery, and then yet again rearranged my schedule during radiation treatment. Again, playing it by ear because I didn't know how I would react to the radiation, I worked a reduced schedule, but came in to the office much more regularly. This year of cancer was stretching the flexibility of my co-workers to the max, but luckily for me, they were up to the task.

After completing all the various cancer treatments, more than nine months from the start, there came again a point in time when I needed to decide how I would continue working. I could have easily slipped back into my old routine of very full-time work, but had discovered over the course of the past nine months that I really liked the freedom of not working full-time. There was something very liberating about having free daytime hours to dream, exercise, cook, meet with friends, play with grandchildren, plan vacations, read, and anything else my little heart desired. I did not want to give up this newfound freedom. I had been toying with the idea of cutting back at work for the last couple of years, but each time the pull of work was too great. There was also the fear of financial insecurity, and the worry that I would cut back days in the office but end up working at home anyway. Although I had known for a while that I wanted to cut back, up until this point I had not been able to extricate myself from the lifestyle and pattern I had developed. Then along came cancer. The cancer wrenched me out of my regular patterns and gave me the chance to take a long, hard look at my life and how I wanted to live it. It was clear to me that cutting back at work was a priority, and cancer definitely paved the way.

As I transitioned back into a stable work pattern, the challenge of organizing the time I have both at work and at home is ever-present. How can I be productive and effective at work, while only dedicating three days a week to this venture? How do I make sure it doesn't creep into my free time as well? The transition to part-time work has not been simple, and there have been bumps in the road. But at the age of 57 I have finally learned to curb my impetuousness, and figured out that sometimes it just pays to sit on things and see what comes next. So, while I haven't figured it all out yet, I am happy with my decision to work fewer days and feel that it is the right decision for me, at this point in time.

TIPS ON WORKING DURING CANCER TREATMENT:

1. Find out what your benefits are, including sick leave, disability insurance, and job security.

2. Have a frank talk with your boss, if possible, letting him or her know that there are many uncertainties in your life and expressing your need for support and flexibility.

3. Understand that your life now is extremely dynamic and unpredictable, and be open to the possibility of change. You may find that you have decided to continue to work, only to find that you simply are not able to keep up physically. On the other hand, you might think that you won't be able to work, and then find yourself bored and wishing you were at work. Be open to change.

4. Prioritize and delegate work tasks for which you are responsible. You will not be able to do it all no matter how hard you try. You also need to take care of yourself.

5. Use this time as an opportunity to explore your feelings about work.

[12]

Complementary Medicine

Update #14 - November 25

As many of you know, I have been interested and involved in alternative therapies for a variety of mild ailments over the years. This certainly has been an opportunity to pull out all the stops and try many different treatments. What I find interesting is that one never knows what exactly is helping, or doing the trick, but I have no doubts that each piece of my treatment plan helps. So what does my week of complementary medicine look like?

The following fills my week:

- *Acupuncture with a specialist in Chinese medicine*

- *13Shiatsu massage (at the Yuri Stern Center – a non-profit center that provides reduced fee treatment for cancer patients and their families)*

- *Llymphatic drainage*

- *Regular massage.*

As you can see – this truly is a full time job! I have no doubts whatsoever that it all has helped me get through these 16 weeks of intense chemo. Additional pieces that have been invaluable to my mind:

- *My daily walk*

- *Guided imagery(bless you Belleruth Naparstek of www.healthjourneys.com)*

- *Learning and reading Psalms*

- *Prayer*

- *Religious study*

- *Even a visit to a kabbalistic rabbi*

I guess I believe in leaving no stone unturned, and have used this challenge as an opportunity to explore things that I might not have otherwise. The acupuncture is the only thing that is occasionally uncomfortable – all the rest feels great - immediately - but I am so convinced of the acupuncture's healing properties that I go along with it happily.

Complementary medicine played a significant role in my healing process. Defining complementary medicine can be tricky, but when I use the term I am referring to a diverse group of medical and health care systems, practices and products that are generally not considered part of conventional medicine. Conventional or Western medicine is practiced by the holder of a medical degree (M.D. or O.D.). Practitioners of complementary medicine vary widely in terms of their training and medical background, thus making the field often confusing to navigate.

Turning to complementary medicine was a very natural response to being diagnosed with cancer for me, as over the years I have dabbled in and tried a variety of complementary medicine treatments for assorted minor ailments. Probably my first encounter with complementary medicine was through Jim Gordon, M.D., a Harvard trained psychiatrist, founder and director of the Center for Mind Body Medicine in Washington D.C. He had come to Israel several years previously to train a group of mental health professionals, of which I was privileged to be part of, in "Mind-Body" Groups and introduced us to the wonderful world of complementary medicine.

Since that time, a decade ago, shiatsu, massage, yoga and meditation have been part of my world. Nevertheless, turning to complementary medicine to help treat cancer may seem to create possible conflict with the fact that I live with my husband, a very conventional doctor practicing conventional medicine. It was not at odds in the least.

Let me stress that what we are discussing here is complementary medicine, in contrast to alternative medicine. The terms complementary and alternative often get mixed up but there is a big difference between the two. Complementary medicine lives in relative peace alongside conventional medicine and is practiced in conjunction with standard, allopathic medicine, not instead of it. Alternative medicine, on the other hand, usually refers to a treatment protocol that takes the place of conventional medicine, going against the better judgment of medical doctors, accepted medical practice and scientific research. Having been married to a medical doctor for 36 years, it was clear to me that conventional medicine was the route I would take. I never even entertained the notion of refusing the conventional treatment offered to me, consisting of surgery, chemo and radiation. I did, however, intend to actively engage in my healing while undergoing many of these procedures, and complementary medicine helped me do that. I was eager to incorporate as much complementary medicine as I could into my treatment to help mitigate the side effects of chemo, and generally strengthen my body and soul and keep me in good shape for the "day after." In addition, complementary medicine allowed me to feel active in my healing process, as opposed to being a passive patient.

A word on control, choice and action is in order here. When I was diagnosed with cancer, it happened to me. I did not choose it. I began my trek from specialist to specialist, test to test, in an attempt to determine what I had and how to best treat it. I was told what to do, where to go, and what treatments I would need. When one becomes a patient there is a certain passivity that takes over, and an overwhelming feeling of loss of control. Deciding to seek out complementary medicine felt to me like I was taking a more active interest in my life and regaining some of that lost sense of control.

When I visited the oncologist and got the news that I would need chemo, I was already actively practicing both guided imagery and yoga. The oncologist mentioned that many people found
acupuncture to be helpful in dealing with some of the side effects of chemo, and I quickly signed on.

For those of you who may be unfamiliar with the world of complementary medicine, a few words on each of the types of treatment that I employed may be helpful here. I should note that there are many additional kinds of treatment, but the ones I chose were fairly mainstream and readily available in my community.

Acupuncture

Acupuncture originated in China and treats patients by inserting thin needles into points in the skin. According to traditional Chinese medicine, stimulation of these points corrects imbalances in the flow of qi (sometimes called chi) or life force. For the first-time patient it can seem a little bizarre, but you quickly get used to lying still for about thirty minutes with needles sticking out of you. After my first chemo treatment I felt simply awful, and I was grateful that the acupuncturist was willing to come to my home to give me a treatment. I immediately felt a lot better after that first treatment, and, from that moment on, I was a convert. I went religiously to my weekly appointment and occasionally, if I was having an especially bad reaction, I would go for an additional treatment. I am certain that the acupuncture had a very important role to play not only in mitigating the side effects of cancer treatment but also in elevating my mood and supporting my overriding sense of balance and ease in the world. I continued acupuncture weekly throughout both chemo and radiation. In my new phase of transition to post-cancer life, I have been exploring the frequency of treatment that feels right to me, as it is clear to me that I want this to remain a part of my wellness routine.

Massage – Conventional and Shiatsu

There are many different schools of massage ranging from Swedish to Thai, Shiatsu to Tuina. Massage has an important place in complementary medicine and it is not difficult to convince most people that massage is good for them. Most people I know enjoy receiving a massage and find it an extremely pleasant experience. I have always been a big fan of massages. I am lucky enough to have a son who is a massage therapist. Wanting to be supportive of him is a good excuse to include weekly massage as part my self-care regimen. That's what you call a win-win. On my first day of chemo, I was pleasantly surprised to find that there were volunteer massage therapists just waiting to work on me in the day treatment center where I received my chemo. While chemo is certainly no treat, this helped to pass the time in a pleasant way and felt very loving and supportive.

Shiatsu massage, like acupuncture, is founded on the Chinese meridian system and it provides a nice adjunct to acupuncture. A shiatsu masseuse first makes his or her diagnosis, assessing where chi (qi) flows freely and where it may be obstructed. The masseuse gently but firmly applies pressure using his or her fingers, knuckles, thumbs, palms, toes, feet, knees, and elbows. Most people find this a pleasurable experience. As I developed a plan for complementary medicine for myself I added shiatsu into the program on a weekly basis and found it gentle and relaxing. I was always left with a sense of wellbeing at the conclusion of treatment.

Nutrition

Nutrition is something that takes center stage in complementary and alternative medicine and occupies many cancer patients in one way or another. Often people undergoing chemo will have side effects that impact upon their appetite and eating. There is also a tremendous amount of information available on the net and the print media about what one should or should not eat. There are schools of thought in which there is a belief that cancer can be cured by diet alone. There are those who think that perhaps our Western diet is one of the root causes of cancer.

The idea that food is medicine is not a new one, but it is gaining acceptance worldwide, even in circles of conventional medicine. Dr. Andrew Weil, an M.D. who has brought the field of complementary medicine into the mainstream, has written extensively about this. Dr. Jim Gordon, a personal friend of mine, has been running "Food as Medicine" conferences for the last number of years. Both practitioners underscore something Maimonides, a great Jewish physician and scholar from the eleventh century, taught us about walking the middle path. While there are nutritional extremists out there, both Weil and Gordon are moderates and served as my guides.

I have been interested in nutrition over the year and find the notion of nutritional intervention to create or speed up healing rather convincing. Over the years I have moved away from the typical Western diet, sometimes called, with tongue in check, the SAD (Standard American Diet). I have become largely vegetarian, avoiding most animal-based meals and processed foods, and eating whole grains, fruits and vegetables, and beans and legumes. The SAD has been heavily implicated in many of the physical ills affecting Western society, including cancer. As an American child I, of course, grew up eating white bread, white flour, white sugar and processed foods but have slowly moved away from this way of eating. During my year with cancer I maintained a fairly steady approach to diet, incorporating small changes and tweaking here and there. In general, I tend to be a fairly mainstream person, rarely going to extremes in any direction. The idea of a strictly macrobiotic diet or a completely raw food diet was hard for me to "stomach", even though these are "the" answer to healing cancer in the opinion of some nutritionists. The changes that I did make included largely reducing sugar from my diet (which isn't to say that I don't occasionally indulge, but for the most part I am sugar-free) and reducing (but not eliminating) my gluten consumption.

An additional change that I incorporated into my routine was juicing. Juicing advocates insist that one can get much higher doses of accessible nutrients in juice than in any other food type. I don't know if this is true, but upon finishing chemo, I celebrated by buying a juicer, and have been juicing daily ever since. The juice I make is made up primarily of vegetables with a knob of ginger and a couple of apples added for taste. My experience with juicing has been extremely positive. I like the juice. It feels good to me. I have good energy all day long and I feel like I am doing something very good for my body. On most mornings two cups of juice is my standard breakfast and usually holds me until about eleven o'clock in the morning. I know that in diet, as in all things, I like variety and change, and as long as that variety and change is in the land of healthful alternatives I think I am ok. So although juicing has been good for me until now, I am open to the possibility that this may change for a while, and then change back once again.

Homeopathy

About six weeks after completing chemo, I developed a strep infection, and was feeling very tired and enervated. I couldn't seem to open my eyes and get going in the mornings. I felt that I had joined the geriatric set as I had to plan my days so that there was time for a nap every afternoon. I limited my nighttime activities. I did not like this lifestyle at all, and while I considered that this might be part of the aftereffects of chemo, I was determined to do something about it. I visited the doctor of Chinese medicine who did acupuncture on me and she suggested I speak to her colleague, the homeopath. Homeopathy started in the 19th century and is a practice based on the concept that a disease can be treated with minute doses of the same substance that causes the disease in healthy people. Studies proving the effectiveness of homeopathic medicine have had very mixed results, and the scientific evidence base for homeopathy is rather shaky. However, as in many areas of complementary medicine, people who use homeopathy swear by it. I decided that I had little to lose and made an appointment with the homeopathic doctor who prescribed a one-month long homeopathic cleanse for me. I immediately went out to the pharmacy and ordered the cleanse, which consisted of four small brown bottles, each with its unknown content (unknown to me, at least). I assiduously mixed thirty drops from each of the four bottles into a 750 cc bottle of water daily for one month. I was to drink a third of this concoction at three times over the course of the day. I figured that it could not hurt, but to say I was skeptical would be an understatement. You can imagine my

amazement when after three or four days of drinking the magic elixir, I felt like I was back to my old self. Not back to my old self before strep, but back to my old self before chemo! My energy had returned along with my vitality and the bounce in my step. I no longer needed to carefully plan my days and measure out my energy expenditure. I felt like I had come back from a long journey and was happily back home in my familiar body. What a pleasure! And what a surprise!

Figuring it all out with all of these options vying for my attention, how was I to figure out what to do? How could I navigate this confusing and complicated terrain? I started with guided imagery immediately upon diagnosis and added acupuncture before beginning chemo, however I was feeling both confused and lousy after just one chemo treatment. Should I change my diet? Should I take herbs? Was there something else I could do that would help me? At that point I decided to consult with a doctor trained in both traditional and complementary medicine. I felt he would both support my combined approach and possibly point the way to additional things I could do to help. It was very important to me that the person I chose to consult with would have a firm grounding in traditional Western medicine so that he would not be against the chemo. I found the consultation quite helpful in reducing confusion and helping me proceed on my healing journey. After asking me many questions about my daily regimen, diet, healthcare, and the course of my disease, the doctor helped me organize my approach. He encouraged me to do acupuncture the day before chemo, and shiatsu a day or two after chemo. He strongly suggested that I do both acupuncture and shiatsu weekly and I adopted this regimen immediately. He also encouraged me to continue with guided imagery and yoga, and to continue with my vegetarian diet, focusing on fresh vegetables in particular. Knowing that I had somebody I could consult with about complementary medicine, who was also knowledgeable and appreciative of conventional medicine, was very helpful to me. It was also, I might add, a very expensive consultation. Cost is definitely an issue that must be considered when discussing complementary medicine. While most health insurances and plans cover expenses incurred by conventional medicine, complementary medicine is, for the most part, rarely covered by insurance plans and is very costly. This may make the decision even more difficult. For myself, I decided that I would freely pursue complementary medicine, and if necessary would cut back on other expenses. My healing was a priority and I was convinced that this was a part of it. Fortunately, I had received some insurance money which I had decided to allocate to cover any and all complementary medicine practices that I wanted. This freed me from thinking about the cost of each treatment.

Keep in mind that the categories of treatment that I have listed here is incomplete. I have written about the things that I did and found most helpful. There are many additional kinds of therapies including energy healing, reflexology, and much more. It is important to explore what works for you and to pursue that. For me, after trying reflexology and energy healing once or twice, and not finding them beneficial to me, I moved on. This is not to say that they would not be helpful to you. The treatments I have included are what worked for me.

Tips on Using Complementary Medicine:

1. Consider adding complementary medicine to your regimen of conventional medicine.

2. Look at your options, see what appeals to you and consider what you can afford.

3. If you can consult with a physician who integrates both conventional and complementary care, this may be very helpful.

4. When trying out new approaches, give them some time, but feel free to stop or change if they don't agree with you. For example, I tried both healing and reflexology and didn't like them that much, so I did not pursue them further.

5. Listen to friendly advice, but remember, once again, that you are unique, and choose what is right for you.

Guided Imagery and Meditation

Update #7 - July 28

So now we have two weeks or so of waiting for the results and the rest of the treatment plan. I fear my updates will get rather boring in the next week or two. I am reading a couple of good novels, doing some writing, a lot of guided imagery (bless your heart, Belleruth), and some good rounds of Connect Four and Mancala with my grandsons.

Remember that image I drew of myself immediately after being diagnosed with cancer? I pictured myself as the helpless kid in that game we used to play as children; I felt like I had been blindfolded and spun around again and again until I was dizzy and confused. In real life, as in the game, it takes a while to regain one's balance. After my shaky footing began to fade, I did remember that I had some landmarks in my life prior to the cancer diagnoses that were ready and waiting for me at this moment of crisis. What were they? Guided imagery and meditation.

Let me backtrack for a moment. I have spent the last ten years working in the field of resilience building with people who have been exposed to trauma. The world of mind-body medicine has informed the programs that we have developed and implemented with educators and first responders in Israel and worldwide. Relaxation, guided imagery, self-hypnosis, mindfulness, and meditation have all been an integral part of these programs as well as a part of my personal life over the last decade. I needed no convincing about the efficacy of these various techniques and practices in reducing stress and promoting healing. It was clear to me that my stress level was high. I was anxious, my sleep was very restless and disturbed, and I felt like my life was totally out of kilter.

What could I do to help myself? I decided that guided imagery was a good way to start. I vividly recall coming downstairs early the morning after having received the grim news and logging onto my computer. Within minutes I had downloaded a guided imagery script on healing cancer created by Belleruth Naparstek (www.healthjourneys.com), a master teacher and trainer in guided imagery. I had been fortunate in meeting her several years earlier in a professional capacity. The download was a true godsend those first few days and weeks after diagnosis. I found that after sixteen minutes a day of guided imagery (and often 32 or 48 minutes, as I listened to the scripts again and again), I was granted a reprieve from worry, feeling relaxed and confident. The soundtracks had the magical ability to make me feel both safe, and at the same time, in control of this situation, two feelings that generally do not go hand in hand with cancer.

So, what is guided imagery? In Belleruth Naparstek's words, "Guided imagery is a gentle but powerful technique that focuses and directs the imagination. It can be just as simple as an athlete's

10-second reverie, just before leaping off the diving board, imagining how a perfect dive feels when slicing through the water. Or it can be as complex as imagining the busy, focused buzz of thousands of loyal immune cells, scooting out of the thymus gland on a search and destroy mission to wipe out unsuspecting cancer cells."

Why does guided imagery work? Guided imagery uses our imaginations in a positive way. My imagination had been working overtime, but in a negative direction. I was imagining my illness, my demise, my funeral and all the rest. What guided imagery helped me do was to direct this very natural and human   activity   called "imagining" into positive and healing channels. When the mind creates images, they can seem almost real. Real tears came to my eyes as I imagined my funeral on that long drive home after receiving the diagnosis. Now, how would I feel if I pictured myself healing? The body responds to images almost as if they are actual events. If we imagine food, we begin to salivate. If I could imagine a safe and beautiful place filled with people who loved me and were sending me good wishes, would I feel safe and cared for? You bet.

The effectiveness of guided imagery has been increasingly established over the last twenty-five years. Studies have demonstrated a positive impact on health, creativity and performance. Blood pressure, cholesterol and glucose levels all show a decline after doing guided imagery. Studies have shown that people who do guided imagery before surgery have reduced blood loss after surgery. While not all these studies conform to the rigorous gold standard of double blind randomized experiments, the evidence is mounting that when the mind thinks positive, something happens in the body, and that something is positive as well. Most important for me was the research showing that guided imagery can help reduce the adverse side effects of chemotherapy, especially nausea, depression and fatigue.

While we have focused here on guided imagery, it is only one of the methods within the mind-body medicine world utilized for stress reduction and wellness. Other approaches include various relaxation and breathing techniques, meditation, mindfulness, yoga, tai chi, Qi Gong and more. Fortunately, I had delved into many of these practices and was familiar with them, so why did I choose specifically to start with guided imagery now? My choice was a considered one, even though it was hasty. I turned to guided imagery because I just knew that I would not have the ability to sit on a meditation cushion, clear my thoughts and breathe at this point in time. My life was racing out of control. My thoughts and emotions flooded my mind and my body felt wired and alien. Clearing my mind seemed to be an impossibility. In contrast, the clear, loving direction in guided imagery directing me, and telling me what to do – how to breathe, what to think, and what to imagine – was very appealing. Belleruth, in her beautiful calm voice accompanied by a ribbon of tranquil music in the background, actively engaged my brain with calming and healing thoughts, so that the maelstrom I found myself in could take a rest. Within a few days of downloading the scripts, merely putting the earphones in my ears and settling down on my bed were cues for the relaxation response to begin. It was remarkable. I began to look forward to my guided imagery sessions as the single oasis in my day where I could take a refreshing pause.

In addition to giving me a sense of calm and safety, the guided imagery focused on healing the cancer. I knew in a very concrete way that I was actively doing something to help heal myself, and while I am a skeptic by nature, and don't really know if guided imagery can cure cancer, I felt that it unequivocally helped me to feel more relaxed, in control, optimistic, and refreshed. It was a true lifesaver and, considering my situation at the time, that is saying quite a lot!

My initial forays into guided imagery focused on healing the cancer. As my treatments progressed, I moved on to guided imagery that focused on healing from surgery, then chemo and finally radiation. I corresponded with Belleruth, who very generously sent me additional downloads and suggested varying what I was listening to from time to time, trying out new voices, different music, and alternate scripts. Somehow, though, I always came home to Belleruth Naparstek. Her voice, her scripts, and her music resonated in a very deep place inside of me. I made sure to take my audio player with me to the hospital and did guided imagery immediately before and after surgery. I took it with me to each chemo session at the day treatment center and listened while the drugs were doing their work. I took it with me to radiation, and listened during many of my radiation treatments. Guided imagery was my trusted partner from start to finish, and one of the cornerstones of my healing regimen.

Other techniques that may be helpful in quieting a feverish mind or a stressed-out cancer patient include mindfulness, meditation, breathing (such as yogic breathing) and Qi Gong. These are all gentle, require minimal physical ability, and can help reduce the anxiety and stress that are prevalent during cancer diagnosis and treatment.

It is important for me to restate the obvious. Guided imagery worked for me. It may be helpful to you, but it may not be. Each person needs to find what is right for them. Because it is easily available, doesn't hurt, and doesn't require a great investment of either money or time, I highly recommend giving it a try if you are on this healing journey, or accompanying somebody along the road.

TIPS ON USING GUIDED IMAGERY AND RELAXATION:

1. If you have never used relaxation or guided imagery before, give it a try. Cancer shakes things up, and provides opportunities to try new things.

2. Find a quiet place and listen to a streaming relaxation guide or MP3 download. Belleruth's website www.healthjourneys.com is a great place to start.

3. Don't expect magic; just expect to feel a bit more relaxed at the start. It often takes several sessions until you get the hang of it.

4. Try other forms of relaxation, meditation or gentle exercise that you think may suit you. Remember – these are things that you can do for yourself that will make you feel better and more in control.

[14]

Fears

Update # 13 – September 27

A friend of mine asked me the other day about the down side of cancer – the worries, the anxieties, the fears, the dark clouds. She remarked that I sound so upbeat that she wondered if these negative feelings even exist for me. I thought to myself that perhaps I am doing an injustice to all of us cancer folks by making this adventure sound so rosy, maybe even Pollyanna-ish.

So let me reassure you that there are plenty of dark moments, and what I do is let them come, and then let them go. People who are close to me on a daily basis – particularly Mike – see me cry, listen to my kvetching (which goes on for days after chemo), and to my darker thoughts. I try not to spread my dark thoughts around, but keep them close. So yes! The fears are there, and I give in to them, but then they go and leave me in peace, and I can once again focus on the much larger parts of my life that are wonderful, and blessed.

Who is most afraid of cancer? Is it the person who has not yet had cancer or those of us who have been treated for cancer and live with the ever-present possibility of recurrence? A moot question I suppose, but fear is one of the companions I have gotten used to living with. Like heartburn, or gas, fear is like an old friend along for the ride. It was not always this way. When I was first diagnosed with cancer, fear was more like a hideous monster, preying on me at unlikely moments during the day, and most particularly during the wee hours of the night. I often had trouble sleeping. Most nights I was so exhausted from the unceasing round of doctor visits, tests, dealing with insurance bureaucracy and consultations that I fell asleep as soon as my head touched the pillow. But after two or three hours of deep sleep I would wake up and start to toss and turn in a valiant effort to return to unconscious slumber. Finally, when the birds began to sing at daybreak, I allowed myself to call it quits on a night's sleep and get out of bed.

Sleep issues plague cancer patients for a variety of reasons. For many, the discomfort associated with treatment may preclude an easy night's sleep. For others, like me, it is the anxieties, the fears, and the worry that keep us up nights. We all know how important and healing a good night's sleep is. But just when you need that most, it escapes you.

For me, the fears that rippled through my sleep and woke me were tangibly claustrophobic. I woke up drenched in sweat. I could not breathe. I was being buried alive. In an alternate dream, I actually was dead yet still gasping for breath. Struggling awake I felt myself choking. While claustrophobia is not new to me, and for years I have refused to crawl through caves, since my regular habitat is above ground this has not bothered me too much nor interfered with my day-to-day life. Now I was panting as I abruptly awakened out of a dream. My logical, daytime mind kept reassuring me that if I was dead I wouldn't need to breathe and that this was really nothing to worry about, but that got me nowhere. Dreams do not usually follow daytime logic. They have a mind of their own. And my mind was overactive and panicky. What to do? I contemplated my options and finally decided to conquer my sleep disturbances by looking the fear of death straight in the eye.

I began to explore a variety of sleeping aids. I decided to try melatonin, a natural drug sold over the counter which is supposed to be a gentle sleeping aid, and is often used to help travelers counteract the effects of jetlag. According to the package instructions, the melatonin might take up to six weeks to work, so I patiently waited for its magic to kick in. After two months of no change I decided to try sleeping pills. I had used sleeping pills occasionally during transatlantic travel and I knew that they would work very well, but I did not like the feeling of being dependent on them. Thus, in the early months after diagnosis, I began to use sleeping pills sporadically, and even then, I would only "allow" myself a half a pill if I was really desperate. As the months of treatment wore on, and the number of medications I was taking increased exponentially due to chemo, I was less resistant to the idea of taking pills and decided to take half a sleeping pill each night, without worrying about dependence and addiction. I would worry about weaning myself off the pills at a later date. What the blessed little pills did was to give me peace of mind and reassurance that I would be able to not only fall asleep but stay asleep, and get at least five or six hours of straight sleep without too many dreams. This was a relief after months of sporadic, fitful sleep filled with tossing, turning and bad dreams.

The third approach I tried to help me overcome sleeplessness was self-hypnosis. This is a form of hypnosis that is self-induced and makes use of suggestions that you give yourself. This technique is sometimes called auto-suggestion. I studied hypnosis many years ago and have used it occasionally in both my professional and personal life, for issues ranging from childbirth and weight loss to test anxiety and snake phobias. I had never used hypnosis for sleep disorders, but then again I had never suffered much from sleep disturbances until this point in time. Hypnosis in general involves an induction phase, which is very similar to inducing a state of deep relaxation. After that, suggestions are introduced. If you want to lose weight the suggestion might be, "I feel full after eating a small amount." If you want to sleep it might be, "I fall asleep easily and wake up fully rested." I set out on a search and easily found some reasonably priced self-hypnosis downloads on the internet that focused on improving sleep. The ones I used were developed by Dr. Steven Gurgevich. I found them relaxing, easy to use and extremely helpful. I was amazed that after doing the self-hypnosis sessions only once or twice my sleep seemed to improve noticeably with or without the sleeping pills.

As the months of treatment wore on, I often listened to the self-hypnosis sleep tapes in the afternoon when I my energies were flagging. I found that listening to them ensured a very deep rest in the afternoon, and I believed that they also improved the quality of my sleep at night. One thing was for sure – it was both easy and painless.

Interestingly, it was important to continue to listen to the tapes on a regular basis for reinforcement. While the cure was not magical, and I sometimes still resorted to using the sleeping pills to help me with the inevitable ups and downs, it seemed to be one more step in the right direction, and one more way that I was able to help myself and take control over my life.

Back to the topic of fears: fears in general and fear of death in particular. (As I write this chapter, I notice how easy it is to digress, and how readily I dove into the side issue of sleep.) Looking back over the year, my fears did not stay the same. They were dynamic and developed and matured over time. After several months, the gasping, choking fears eased and were supplanted by fears of metastases. I couldn't get out of my mind the concern my oncologist had expressed that I was at risk for metastases. My imagination began to run wild. I coughed once and I pictured my lungs riddled with cancer. I was sure the cancer had spread. I had a headache and imagined my brain spotted with the disease. All of this symbolized most clearly to me my fear of death. Here I was looking death squarely in the face. No beating around the bush. Did I want to die? No. Was I ready to die? No. Had anybody said I was going to die now? Also no. I found a great deal of solace in the Buddhist writings of Thich Nhat Hahn, a Buddhist monk whose book Fear Not Death I had acquired and read sporadically over the years. Now each page was more meaningful than ever. Metaphorically holding his hand, I was able to calm down and remember: we all die. Some of us die sooner and others die later. But we all die.

My mind was occupied with thoughts such as, "What is my job here on this earth? Why am I here? What is it I want to be doing with the time I have? Do I want to spend my months and years in fear of the inevitable? How can I live my life in the shadow of death without being paralyzed? How can I use the time that God has given me on this earth to the greatest good?" Thich Nhat Hahn's voice was both reassuring and sane. His teachings in mindfulness helped as I breathed into the moment. I grounded myself in the present. I was here. Now. I was coping. Things were going fairly well. Breathe in. Breathe out.

That worked for a bit, but then my monkey mind began to chatter. Monkey mind is a Buddhist term used by people who meditate to indicate restlessness, an unsettled and confused mental state. Thoughts kept racing around my mind, and especially the thought "mets, mets, mets," (short for metastases, of course).

I had had a bone scan and a CAT scan before chemo began, and everything had checked out clear, so why was I obsessing about metastases? And which metastases? Initially, I was worried about lung metastases because breast cancer often goes to the lungs. That is what you get for being a doctor's wife – you know a little bit about a lot of things. Every time I had a little phlegm in my chest, or a cough, I was sure that was it. I was a goner. I walked around for weeks picturing my slow, withering death. A neighbor of mine, about my age, had recently died from lung cancer, and I knew she had suffered for many long months. I kept these fears to myself for the most part and didn't share them even with those closest to me. Why? My logical mind kept saying, "Don't be a drama queen. Don't be ridiculous. You checked out clean. You are getting chemo. You do not have lung mets. People are going to think you are going crazy." But logic only goes so far here. Eventually, I shared my worries with my husband, who listened carefully and took me seriously. He patiently reassured me that he really, really did not think I had lung metastases.

Eventually that fear receded, only to be supplanted by the fear of brain metastases. During my months of treatment, I had met a woman at one of my treatment appointments who seemed to have a very similar disease course as mine until that point: lumpectomy, chemo, and radiation. We laughed together about how we had used the same surgeon, the same oncologist, the same physiotherapist, and here we were even at the same massage center. She had finished her cancer treatments about six months ahead of me, and was both reassuring and encouraging. She showed me how her hair was growing in and told me how well she was feeling and enjoying life. She was very outgoing and friendly, and we exchanged phone numbers, e-mails, and Facebook names. I began to follow her on Facebook as she took a celebratory trip overseas for a month. When she returned, she not only had terrible jetlag, but a persistent headache that would not go away. Sure enough, within a week of return, she was diagnosed with brain mets, and underwent surgery. I was sure that I was next up. My identification with her was so great that it was hard for me to separate my story from hers. My heart pounded as I scanned Facebook daily and sometimes hourly for messages from her. I desperately wanted to know every detail of her disease, yet at the same time I wanted to deny it all and bury my poor head in the sand. I continued to follow her until the day she stopped writing and I understood that despite her invincible spirit, her body   had succumbed.

My fear of brain mets was so real that I began to experience regular headaches, kind of a zinging that was fairly painful but lasted only a couple of seconds. It was always in the same place. I could localize exactly where the met was! I also experienced dizziness, and a fuzzy feeling of altered consciousness and disconnectedness. Again, I walked around for weeks with fear in my heart and on my mind. My logical brain tried to dismiss the worries, but my heart and soul were sick with them. I finally shared my fears with my husband, and once again he tried to explain to me how the feelings and sensations I was having were most likely not manifestations of a metastasis. He told me that if the symptoms got worse or changed we would have to check them out. I went to my family physician, who listened carefully as I described my symptoms. I greatly appreciated how she was able to listen to me, take me seriously and not dismiss my distress as "all in my head." Upon completing a thorough physical and neurological exam, she said that I had nothing but a bad case of the "wobbles" which I was certainly entitled to, considering all I had been through over the past months, including surgery and chemo. Amazingly, my headaches cleared up almost completely within a week or two of visiting her and being diagnosed with the wobbles. Once again, the mind-body connection was reaffirmed. The way my imagination could be used for positive healing on the one hand, and yet run wild and convince me that I was deathly ill, was remarkable.

The mild dizziness and feelings of disconnect accompanied me much longer, and I decided that this was my form of "chemo brain" and something I could learn to live with much more easily if I didn't panic about it. When I discussed my symptoms with my oncologist, he offered to do a CAT scan of my head. Although he did not feel it was necessary or recommend it, he offered it as a way of giving me peace of mind. I decided to wait a month and if I did not improve, I would schedule the test. Fortunately, within the month I felt much better and did not do the scan.

Does that mean that all my fears have receded for good? By all means, no! They are, however, less acute and I am preoccupied with them much less of the time. On good days I am able to label my fears and say, "Oh, there are the cancer fears," and somehow that minimizes them and makes them recede. Labeling the fears helps me to normalize them and give them boundaries. I have also learned the importance of getting symptoms checked out even if they are "all in my head." And one last thing I have learned is that it is not good, I repeat, NOT GOOD, to keep these fears to myself. When I keep these fears to myself they only thrive and grow and steal away my joie de vivre and sense of balance. Sharing them with others brings them out into the light of day, where they can shrivel up and disappear, and leave me free to lead my life fully, happily and for the most part anxiety-free.

Without a doubt, one of the very biggest challenges of transitioning back into life after completing cancer treatment is learning how to manage these fears and recognize them as one of the permanent features of my personal landscape. My fears have become more comfortable and less scary, reminding me of an old pair of shoes that I really don't need anymore, but have a hard time giving up because we have been through so much together.

TIPS ON MANAGING FEARS:

1. Acknowledge your fears to yourself.

2. Talk about your fears with a close friend or partner.

3. If you feel that your fears are getting the better of you, seek professional help. This is an area where there are tried and true solutions waiting for you.

4. Check out physical symptoms with your physician. Do NOT be embarrassed to bring up any worries or concerns you may have. This is their job.

5. Try self-hypnosis or relaxation tapes if (when) your sleep is disturbed.

6. Breathe into the moment. Breathe in. Breathe out. Focus on your breath. Notice it going in. Notice it going out. All we have is this moment. All we have is the present. It is a present (corny but true). Smile.

[15]

Faith, Spirituality and Eating on Yom Kippur

A diagnosis of cancer can put you on the fast track to spiritual adventure. Why me? Why now? What is God trying to tell me? Questions like these made their appearance within the first hour of receiving my diagnosis. I quickly pushed those existential – and to my mind, unanswerable – questions aside. Rather than delve into "why me?" I chose to focus on figuring out what the purpose of this disease was for me, in my life, now. What was I to do with this cancer? What could I make of it? What significance and meaning could I build around it?

Meaning and significance play an important part in the resilience-building model that I work with professionally in my capacity as a trauma psychologist. From my experience, I know that when people can find meaning in difficult situations they fare much better. They often come out of a traumatic encounter with renewed strength and what we psychologists call "post-traumatic growth." At this moment in time I was not concerned with how the search would play out in my life and what the net results of my search for meaning would be. This search felt like an instinctual drive similar to what Viktor Frankl discusses in his classic book, Man's Search for Meaning, in which he discusses how man can tolerate just about everything if he has a "why", a reason to live for. For me, this search for meaning was not so much a conscious choice, but more of a response to an inborn need. When talking about searching for meaning it should be noted that the search, in and of   itself,   is important. Whether one ever finds the definitive answer is almost irrelevant. For most of us there probably is not one answer.

So searching for meaning was clearly on the table. For me, the natural direction pointed to religious sources and inspiration. Having grown up in traditional Judaism, I was not a stranger to thinking about God in a personal, relational sort of way, despite the fact that for me He (She?) had been benevolently remote as a child and through my young adulthood. In recent years, my newfound emotional and spiritual connection to Jewish practice has grown and has joined the older, well-worn intellectual avenues with which I grew up. While my relationship to God has had its ups and downs, over the years it has become more familiar and intimate.

Part of that intimate relationship revolves around daily prayer, a cornerstone of Jewish practice. Prayer has been a relatively constant part of my life, to a greater or lesser degree, for as long as I can remember. I grew up in a family that attended synagogue regularly and emphasized the importance of prayer. More recently, spending time studying religious texts has taken center stage in my spiritual practice. When I received the diagnosis of cancer, I was spending about one hour a day studying Talmud, the canonical body of Jewish law and lore. I would wake up early in the morning to have a clear, fresh mind for this very intensive and exacting study, and would pore over the page of small print written in ancient Aramaic. After being diagnosed with cancer, I struggled for the clarity and single-mindedness I had found in Talmud study, but within a few weeks, I felt vanquished. I just could not concentrate or muster the energy to focus. I simply did not have the tremendous willpower it took to continue this practice that I had been doing for the last four years. The intellectual effort became overwhelming for me, and upon deciding to let it go I felt a mingled sense of relief, sadness and disappointment.

Now that I was no longer studying Talmud on a daily basis I felt a huge gap open up in my life, both in terms of freeing up a daily hour of time as well as a lacuna in my relationship with God. I was used to encountering God every morning in the pages of the Talmud. I often found myself carrying on a dialogue with Him and with the great Sages of the Talmud. What would take the place of this important pursuit? I knew that I wanted to continue some kind of daily textual study, as it gave me a structure that I found helpful. If I were to leave things to chance or whim, I would probably not get around to studying or talking to God very often. I fortuitously decided to study the Book of Psalms, choosing a chapter a day as my focus. According to tradition, King David wrote most of the Psalms and over the millennia, it has been the go-to book for people in trouble. Many chapters of Psalms have been incorporated into the daily Jewish prayer. However, I had never studied the Psalms as a corpus on its own. The texts themselves are much more straightforward than those in the Talmud and much shorter, as well. After some deliberation, I decided to fill my early morning study hour with a chapter a day from the Book Of Psalms. In this way, I calculated, I would finish the entire book by the end of chemo. This was certainly a less

demanding goal than continuing with my daily Talmud study and I thought that the timing was very neat. Unfortunately, my calculations were (perhaps not surprisingly, considering my chemo brain) in error and despite my daily study, I had many chapters to complete in the Book of Psalms long after chemo was completed. This proved not to be a problem because by then I was hooked and totally under the thrall of this remarkable book. As the Psalms began to weave their magic I was amazed to discover how each and every chapter seemed to be talking directly to me in a very personal and profound way. I knew that the Psalms were written specifically for me and for what I was going through. I felt embraced and enveloped by the Psalms; I felt understood. I felt that God was listening to me in my plight.

My practical nature had steered me toward the question of what TO DO with the cancer, rather than the unanswerable "why me?" However, the "why me?" question did not go away and I ultimately decided to pay attention. The discussion inside my head went something like this: "This is futile! Do you really expect to find a clear answer? Is there an answer? Could there be an answer? Will asking this question lead me down the thorny path of guilt and a detailed list of past sins? How will that help me?" So many questions. It felt like a swarm of bees circling my head. Maybe it would be better to lay this seemingly futile search to rest, to step aside and let the bees find a more hospitable hive. There was no guarantee that I would find honey at the end of the road, and more likely I would be stung. Unhappily, I found that I was unable to put the issue to rest, as the questions just kept coming right back at me. I realized I had no choice but to look these difficult questions square in the face.

I knew this was a road that I should not walk alone. I decided to approach several people with my questions. Some of them were acknowledged spiritual leaders, others were people who seemed to me to be kind and wise. I was pleasantly surprised that   these conversations were welcomed, and that the folks with whom I had chosen to talk this over were no strangers to these types of conversations and discussions.   The answers I received were as varied and different as their personalities and their life circumstances, although all assured me that this was a legitimate course of pursuit. Not one of them said to me, "Drop it."

One of the pearls I received during this time was from an elderly gentleman who shared with me something that he had heard many years earlier from his very well-known teacher. He told me that God might one day whisper in my ear and tell me what this is all about. But then again, he cautioned, He might not. If God does whisper in my ear, perhaps I will hear him but then again, maybe I won't. In any case, this wise man assured me, I am the only one who will know whether God has appeared to me, and I am the only one that will hear what He is saying. This man's message to me was that it certainly was nobody else's business to tell me: "This is what you have done wrong!" I found his words both comforting and encouraging. In retrospect, trying to figure out why this was so helpful to me, I think that what I took away from the encounter was the encouragement to continue developing a close, intimate relationship   with   a   very particular God with whom I could find comfort and solace, rather than walk down the dark, lonely avenues of despair.

The backdrop to many of these discussions was the Jewish High Holiday season which quickly approached as I had completed two rounds of chemo and was adjusting to my new reality of bi-monthly chemo treatments. The Jewish High Holidays are a time for introspection and a spiritual accounting of one's life and one's actions in the past year. In Israel at this time of year, the whole country seems to be caught up in an examination of the good life, the moral, ethical and meaningful life that is worth living. My personal quest fit right in to the spirit of the times. By the time the Jewish New Year arrived, I had crossed the line and I both looked and felt like a cancer patient. The bald head was a giveaway, but I was also feeling the aftereffects of chemo. I applied and received a permit for my car to allow me to park in handicapped spots. I could legally buy medical marijuana. These were some of the trappings of my new status. Crossing over this line also meant that I was going to eat on Yom Kippur, the Day of Atonement, the holiest day of the year. Since I was twelve years old I have fasted the 25 hours of Yom Kippur, abstaining from both food and drink for that period of time. I could never have imagined in my wildest dreams actually eating and drinking on Yom Kippur. I have mentioned earlier the feeling of crossing the line between the world of the living and healthy, and the world of the sick. There are different lines to consider crossing as well. For example, there are the social lines: I am sick you are not. There are lines that are physical such as you feeling well and I don't, you having hair while I don't. Then there are the spiritual lines. While fasting on Yom Kippur, the solemnest day on the Jewish calendar, seems like something physical, in fact the line that I was crossing on that day was a spiritual one in its very essence. My oncologist had told me, in no uncertain terms, that fasting on Yom Kippur was forbidden for me this year. As a matter of fact, he said that it was a mitzvah (a positive commandment) for me to actually eat on Yom Kippur. I of course checked this out with my local rabbi, who concurred completely. I was most definitely forbidden to fast on this Yom Kippur and was required to eat and drink. How was I going to do this? I could not imagine it. While my head understood logically that this year was not a year to fast, my soul felt ostracized. I had stepped beyond the pale, into another space, and was not part of the community. It was clear to me that I would have to use mind over matter in order to get through this most unusual Day of Atonement.

As I contemplated eating on Yom Kippur this year, the year of my cancer, the High Holidays took on a new dimension of meaning. "Who will live and who will die?" is one of the central prayers of the day, and the theme that serves as the subtext for the entire month leading up to the pinnacle, which is Yom Kippur. The entire Jewish People were caught up in the same questions that were wracking my brain and body. Only this time I knew that my life was really on the line. I felt that I could take the lead in crying out this prayer for the entire community, but how could I do that and then go home to eat? It felt like a contradiction in terms. In fact, it was a contradiction in terms, but to me that is the beauty of my Judaism which encompasses diversity, opposing positions, and the ebb and flow of life. Here in a nutshell was that dynamic: first a prayer from the heart pleading for health and life, and then breaking one of the most cardinal of Jewish laws by going home to eat, on this holiest of days, Yom Kippur.

And that is exactly what I did. While I ate and drank normally throughout the evening and the day, I made sure not to eat in front of family members who were, of course, fasting. In preparing for this day, I thought about the prayers that would accompany this eating. I created special blessings to sanctify the wine. I broke bread using two loaves, the way we do every

Friday night, because Yom Kippur is the Sabbath of all Sabbaths. I added holiday prayers in the Grace After Meals, and I felt deep in my heart that this Yom Kippur was a very special one because I, and only a few select others, were able to make these unusual blessings. I was surprised how once I started drinking and eating, it seemed completely normal, and not at all unusual. As so often happens, the anticipation and build up were much more significant than the event itself. The idea of eating on this solemn fast day turned out to be much harder than the eating itself.

In conclusion, while this may be a truism or obvious, spiritual succor had a substantial place in my year of healing from cancer. I found avenues of prayer and study in my native traditional Judaism that fed my need to feel held in the hand of a personal God; one who cared about me and was watching over me. From the Buddhist tradition I took the skill and practice of mindfulness, the acute awareness of the transitory nature of time and the understanding that we will all die someday. In guided imagery I was able to conjure an image of me resting in the palm of God's hand. All of this blended together, creating for me a strong and positive spiritual presence during this most trying of years.

TIPS ON LEADING A SPIRITUAL LIFE DURING CANCER:

1. Cancer is a time to enrich your spiritual life and practice.

2. If you already have a spiritual practice be open to modifying it in order to adjust to both your physical and emotional needs.

3. If you have never considered yourself a spiritual person, now is the time to explore.

4. Avail yourself of spiritual guides, support, hospital chaplains, religious leaders and others who can provide support of a different sort than the medical professionals.

5. Explore new and alternative forms of spiritual practice including meditation, poetry, the arts and anything else, which might serve you as an avenue of connection to "the great beyond."

6. Engage family and friends in existential discussions. You are right now in the eye of the proverbial storm, and they may be thankful for your opening up a topic about which they too have been thinking.

7. Understand that spirituality plays an important role in the healing journey and allow space and time for it in your life.

[16]

Taking a Vacation from Cancer

Update #17 - January 8

The last you heard from me, Mike and I were off to vacation in the North. We wanted to squeeze it in between completing chemo and my second surgery. We had a wonderful time at a small B&B. The view was so amazing – the entire wall of the cabin was one big window — that we hardly wanted to go anywhere. We pulled ourselves away to visit a winery, an olive press, a cheese farm (we ate well), and to go to our favorite sulfur springs. All in all, it was a great vacation and a wonderful break from the everyday routine.

How can you take a vacation from cancer? Is that legal? Is it allowed? For me, sneaking in mini-vacations every chance we got was a wonderful break from both the day-to-day grind, as well as a chance to almost (but not quite) forget that I had the big C. Getting away allowed me to feel normal and to step out of my role as "the sick one" for just a little while. It was a huge relief to focus on what we were going to do that day, where we would eat, and how we would enjoy ourselves, instead of weighing the pros and cons of mastectomy versus lumpectomy, or anticipating chemo. Being in surroundings where people did not know me, and did not know that I had cancer, reminded me of what life was like without cancer. I didn't have to deal with the searching looks, the interested questions, and the constant caring, which despite being well-meaning and supportive did cast me in the role of cancer patient. The opportunity to glimpse beyond all that, and to remember for even a day or two what is was like to be just a regular person, was a wonderful relief.

Vacation was not only good for me, it was also important for my dedicated spouse. Mike certainly deserved a vacation as well. Not only did he have to deal with his sick wife, he was also mourning the loss of his father. During this entire year the focus was on me and Mike was entirely dedicated to whatever I wanted and what I needed. Going on vacation gave a little attention to his needs as well. It also gave us time to be together as a couple, something that very often got lost in the shuffle.

Perhaps this is a good place to touch upon the tricky subject of intimate relationships and cancer. Cancer is definitely a major stressor. Research and life experience has taught us that couples that are doing poorly as a couple before cancer knocks on their door will find that cancer does not improve their relationship. There are stories out there about cancer patients whose spouses have deserted them during cancer treatment. There are other stories of cancer patients who have decided to leave their spouses either before or after treatment. It is almost as if they are saying – life is too short to live it in this unhappy relationship.

Even the best of relationships will undergo a battering during cancer. One part of the couple has all of a sudden become much needier. The needs may be physical, they may be economic, but they are always emotional. Intimate relationships provide a unique kind of support that cannot be replaced. If the healthy spouse is not able to come through with this support, this may prove to be a big disappointment. On the other hand, if the healthy spouse is able to gather his or her own personal resources and be there for their sick partner, this can be a time when a relationship becomes much closer, more loving, and more focused on the positive.

I was fortunate (what an inadequate word!) to find myself in just such a relationship. I have mentioned that my spouse is a physician, and as such he was able to help me navigate the medical world. But in addition to that, he was 100% there for me and able to support me through the rough times. Often I would catch him looking at me with loving eyes, with a look that I had never quite seen or noticed before. It was as if he was no longer taking my presence for granted, and was treasuring every moment we had. This feeling of being thankful for what we had shared until now and reveling in the moment, because who knew what the future would bring, was very poignant and loving.

Most of our lives together (and we have been married for well over thirty-five years) we negotiate and compromise and decide what we will do, where we will go, what we will eat, etc. etc. All of a sudden, Mike was deferring to me. Whatever I wanted to do was what we did. Wherever I wanted to go was where we went. It was as if he had made a conscious decision that this year of cancer treatment, no matter what, we would not fight or argue over the little piddly things that had been a regular feature on the landscape of our relationship. When we had our first fight, many months after I completed cancer treatment, I laughed to myself and was actually relieved. I now knew for sure that I was healthy again, and things were moving back to normal.

Back to vacations. The vacations we took were obviously dictated by both my current physical state at the time, and when the next treatment was set to begin. Thus, while we might have wished to take a month-long trek in Nepal, we were limited to two or three day getaways not too far from home. We tended to choose places that were pampering, and decided on activities that were restful, relaxing and non-demanding. This suited both of us and still gave the feeling of having gotten away, and an opportunity to refresh and recharge batteries. Planning the vacations when I was recuperating from either surgery or chemo gave me a sense of perspective. It also opened up vistas far beyond my bed or the sofa where I tended to spend most of my hours on bad days. In our family, I tend to be the one to plan vacations, but I usually do it at Mike's behest – so it really is a combined effort, and we usually are both in agreement when it comes to getting away.

For those people for whom a few days away seems an impossibility, whether due to financial constraints or family responsibilities, a night out can do the trick as well. The idea is to allow yourself a break from the constant worry of cancer and – if you have a spouse or partner and are doing it with him or her – a chance to grow your relationship. A movie and dinner out will provide enough of a distraction to help you forget cancer for a few moments or a few hours. If you are going out with a friend or relative, you can lay the ground rules that the subject of cancer is "out of bounds" and that you want to forget it for a few hours. If a movie and dinner are not your style, take a drive out to the country, go shopping, or pay a visit to a museum. Do something that you like and, if you have a partner, do something that you both enjoy. By allowing yourself a mini-vacation from daily drudgery and responsibilities, you will return refreshed and with more resolve to beat that cancer.

Tips for Vacationing during Cancer:

1. Schedule short vacations when your treatment schedule allows for it.

2. Even a day or two away can feel like a refreshing break from the daily grind.

3. If you can, spoil yourself and choose vacations where you feel pampered.

4. Enjoy nature or activities that you have enjoyed in the past.

5. Use this time to explore new places and activities, but keep it simple and close to home. This reduces the effort in planning and getting there and allows for more flexibility – which you may need during treatment, when you are not quite sure how you will feel.

6. Vacationing with spouse or children is a good way to make them feel remembered and appreciated during a time when they are often overlooked and overworked.

[17]

Radiation

I am sitting here in front of Room Number 35, in the sub-sub- basement of Hadassah Medical Center in Ein Kerem. I will get to know this place pretty well over the next seven weeks, as I am due to show up here five days a week for a series of 33 radiation treatments. The way I view this phase is that it is a "mop up" operation to catch any stray cancer cells in my breast or chest area. I am not sure that is quite accurate, but that is my view of things. Is it a momentous day? Not really. Many friends have been surprised that I have come here all by myself, without accompaniment, but I didn't feel like I needed anybody along, and felt fine coming here alone. Fortunately for me, Hadassah is close to where I work, about a five-minute drive (not counting parking, of course,) and I am fitting this appointment into a pretty busy day at work. I have had loads of offers to drive me to and from radiation but at this point in time I hope to be able to go and come on my own. The big challenge is the waiting. The way it works is that you come in and sign up, and then wait. It's not clear to me why they don't give you a set appointment. This is kind of like the old-style medicine that was typical forty years ago, when we first moved to Israel. At that time, in all the health clinics, you would come in and take a number and then sit and wait till called. You couldn't make an appointment for a set hour. Sometimes the wait was a few minutes, but more often a few hours. I, of course, will try to finesse the system and figure out when the wait will be the shortest. Already I have chosen well – I asked to be scheduled in the afternoon, figuring that then I won't have to fight morning traffic and crowds. This seems to be true. I even got a parking spot right outside of the building where all cancer treatments take place. Beginner's luck?? Time will tell.

Radiation should be a breeze. Relative, that is, to chemo. Having survived two surgeries and chemo quite well, I was rather cavalier and confident about facing the challenges of radiation. I was set to have a relatively long course of 33 radiotherapy sessions, lasting exactly six and a half weeks. In the area where we live there is only one hospital that has radiotherapy facilities. It was not the hospital that I had become so familiar with over the course of the last few months, the place where I had surgery and chemo. Nevertheless, I was eager to get started as soon as possible so that I could finish the treatments and (hopefully) put this period of my life permanently behind me. I got the green light to start radiation about one month after my second surgery.

The secretary with whom I initially spoke sounded lovely, kind, and interested. What a nice surprise. She scheduled a pre-radiation preparatory appointment for me without delay for early the following week. This seemed promising and I was impressed. It was only when I got to the medical center that the real fun began. First of all, parking was impossible. After finally wrangling a spot, and walking miles through the maze of parking lots, I arrived out of breath but just on time for my appointment. In reality it didn't seem to matter. My 2:30 appointment was apparently a fiction. I had to add my name to a handwritten list and wait. It was first come, first serve. Unfortunately, this was just a little taste of what was to come.

When I finally got in to see the doctor, a lovely young woman, I realized that this was the first female doctor I had seen during my whole experience with breast cancer. I noticed that I liked having a female doctor. Despite the fact that I had been examined what felt like hundreds of times over the year, I was surprised to find that it was easier to bare my breast to a woman. She briefly explained the radiotherapy process to me and scheduled me for a simulation, at which time all the technical aspects of the radiation would be marked off and set up. After that I would be scheduled to begin treatment.

I arrived for my second appointment at the radiotherapy department, after dealing with the rigmarole of parking and what appeared to be the standard long wait time. I was finally ushered into the simulation room, and asked to take off the clothes on the top half of my body. I was then asked to lay down on a cold metal bed in a very cold room with big machines. The efficient and business-like X-ray technician exhorted me not to move AT ALL. Unfortunately, nobody took the time to explain to me what was going to happen or prepare me. The techs went about their business very professionally but with little warmth or caring. Pictures were taken from every angle. People hovered over me, back and forth and back and forth. My breast was painted up in all sorts of weird designs, lines and arrows to mark exactly where the machines needed to be positioned to do their work. My understanding is that in many radiation therapy clinics tattoos are used to help guide the machines. For whatever reason, this advanced medical center still paints what felt like primitive war paint all over my poor breast. During the course of treatment, touchups to the paint were done with permanent markers, but on that first day, the "war paint" was used to mark me up.

When the simulation was finished and I was finally allowed to get up, I felt frozen, both from the cold machinery and from the subzero temperature in the room. My back was totally stiff from lying motionless for an hour, and I was not a happy camper. Before leaving, I was warned not to erase the lines of paint until I began treatment ten days later. When I asked how I was supposed to make sure the lines did not disappear for ten days, the techs told me not to shower on that side. For the next week I lived in dread of disappearing lines, worrying that they would have to repeat the simulation, or that the radiation would be focused on the wrong areas. I wondered to myself why they could not figure out a better method than this one in the 21st century. Moreover, I felt like I was being treated like an object, and not like a person. I missed the warm, supportive atmosphere that I had experienced in the day treatment center where I had received my chemo. What could have been a relatively minor interlude in my life was turning into an unpleasant experience. This only augured what was to come. When I initially went for the simulation, I inquired about which times were the lightest in terms of patient flow, and when I would be able to get in and out as expeditiously as possible. I was totally flexible and was prepared to come first thing in the morning or last thing in the evening. I was told that afternoons were generally lighter, and I was scheduled on a machine that was active both mornings and afternoons. The first day I came in exactly at 2:30. I waited around 45 minutes before I was taken in for treatment. Little did I know that was considered a short wait. For reasons unbeknownst to me, patients were not given exact hours for appointments, and people arrived whenever it was convenient for them. I didn't care what time of day I came. The only thing that was important to me was to spend as little time as possible waiting. Since the department was managed in such a haphazard fashion, this was to prove impossible.

Unfortunately, waiting has never been my strong suit. I am an impatient person by nature and I move quickly, think quickly, and do not suffer waits well. Catch me in a long line at the supermarket and you will find an unhappy person. Traffic jams drive me crazy. I was sure that I would be able to crack the system and find the right time of day to come so that I would have only a short wait. So, I tried 6:30 in the morning. That didn't work. Then I tried later in the day. That didn't work either. No matter when I came, I ended up waiting anywhere between forty-five minutes and three hours. This was not a morale booster, to put it mildly.

I had been forewarned about the long waits in the radiotherapy clinic before I started radiation by a friend who had recently undergone treatment. Knowing my short fuse, and sensing that this was something I would have no control over, I thought that the best way to approach this challenge was to start a writing project. I would write poems, or a journal, or something that I would have to show for all the hours of wait, at the end of the six and a half weeks of daily treatment. In retrospect, the idea of starting a specific project was a good one, but the medium I chose was the wrong one for me. Perhaps if I had chosen a crafts projects I might have been more successful. During much of the wait time I was so antsy and frustrated that I just couldn't concentrate and write. I quickly gave up on this idea and soon I was just trying to pass the time as pleasantly as possible. I brought books, listened to tapes, and talked to other patients. I felt frustrated beyond belief, and I knew that this was not good for my healing. I am a person who likes to make almost every minute of the day count. The waste of time that occurred while waiting for treatment was incredible. Here I was, trying to put my life back together, get back on track, return to work and feel a sense of control over my life, and they seemed to be doing everything in their power to

undermine my efforts. Add to that the number of people who felt really lousy while they were waiting in this dungeon-like atmosphere and you begin to get the dim picture. And I do mean dim.

The radiotherapy department is located two floors underground with no windows, lit by harsh fluorescent lights. As I descended the stairs (I quickly discovered that this was the preferred route and much quicker than waiting for the elevators) I felt like I was entering a dungeon. The hallways were lined with chairs and the chairs were filled with cancer patients awaiting treatment. The patients were of every sort and variety, from people with disfigured faces, missing ears and nose, to people lying in hospital beds groaning. There were even young children being wheeled in for radiation. The exposure to these sights hour after hour, day after day, week after week, had a wearing and dispiriting effect. Add to that the difficulties parking, the long wait, and the frequent machine malfunctions, and you have a recipe for frustration, anger, and despair. Unexpectedly, radiation was becoming much more challenging than the chemo. My spirits were flagging.

The actual radiation treatment itself was usually a relief after the long wait. During the treatments I plugged into my MP3 and listened to guided imagery that was both calming and supportive. I quickly found that there were a few techs I liked, who were kind, respectful and caring, and I tried to come during the hours when they were working. By the end of the 33 treatments I had finally figured out how to finesse the system, but I was worn out and angry from the incredible waste of time, and what felt to me like a colossal lack of respect for the patients and their suffering.

My experience with radiation was similar to that of several of the women whom I had met along the journey. We had all been led to believe that radiation was a piece of cake, when in fact it was much more onerous than expected. In the preparatory meeting before radiation, the side effects that had been discussed included fatigue and possible local skin reactions, particularly burns. I had heard that these burns could be avoided by using special creams. The doctors and techs at the clinic all forbid me from using any creams. However, after consulting with the complementary medicine doctor to whom I had gone months earlier, I slathered myself with a calendula-based cream every evening during the six and a half weeks of radiotherapy. Interestingly, I had no skin reactions until the very last week, when I got burns in two small spots. The burns were painful and annoying – and they were in places that I had missed and had not applied the cream. It took over three weeks for the burns to heal and I was thankful that I had ignored the hospital folks and followed the good advice of my consultant.

As far as fatigue was concerned, right around the time I started radiation I also started a homeopathic cleanse (see Chapter 12). Within three or four days of beginning the cleanse,

I began to feel back to my regular self. Instead of measuring out my activities in small doses and making sure that I would be back home for an afternoon nap, I found that I was able to go out freely, and not worry about when I would be able to get back into bed. Whether it was the homeopathic cleanse or something else at work, I don't know, but I did not suffer from excessive fatigue during the entire course of radiation. I kept waiting for the other shoe to drop, but it never did.

Considering this period of time in hindsight, it is not surprising that my mood was down, to say the least, and it would not be surprising to me if others fellow cancer patients experience a sense of mild depression during this time. By the time I began radiation treatments, cancer was not something new. My adrenalin rush was long gone. It was more of a feeling of "been there, done that", and "let's get on with life". Add to that the frustration of the actual day-to-day functioning of the radiotherapy department and the daily contact with so many others with cancer and you have a recipe for dysphoria. Was there anything else I could have done during this time to help me out of the funk?

One thing I did that I am sure helped was that I kept exercising. There is very good research that shows that exercise is as good as or better than anti-depressant medication. My daily walk was good for my body as well as my soul.

I also think that expectation had a great deal to do with how I was feeling. My expectation of radiation was that it would be a breeze, no big deal. If, in fact, someone had prepared me that, aside from the expected side effects, this might be an especially wearing time, I would have been forewarned possibly protecting myself and shoring myself up better. I guess I felt somewhat broadsided by what was happening. Although I had a lot of support in place and I continued much of the complementary medicine, it did not seem to be enough. Perhaps knowing ahead of time how difficult this time would be emotionally, might have prevented me from dipping so low or been so angry.

Update # 19- March 6

Today is treatment #32, and tomorrow is the day I finish my radiation treatments. So it is time to check in. My sense is that while treatment is ending, the journey is still midway, so you probably will hear from me again. So after treatment #33 is completed, then what?

Life!

The immediate plans are to go away for a week with my steady and devoted walking partner to a health farm (wheat grass, raw food, etc.) for five days to wind down and detox from all these treatments. I look at this as the start of my physical renewal process. A week later I continue the process, going with Mike to Venice and northern Italy for eight nights.

So those are the details – but what is behind those details? Lots of thoughts about how one transitions from active treatment to watchful waiting.

TIPS ON RADIATION TREATMENT:

1. Educate yourself about what to expect. Don't expect the hospital staff will tell you. You will need to ask. Do not be afraid of asking again and again.

2. To people who have been through radiation for specific tips they can offer.

3 .Do something special on the weekends when you can take a break from radiation. Spoil yourself. Treat yourself better than usual. You deserve it. You are almost there.

4. Plan your celebration for completing treatment, down to the details. Use that as a focal point and distraction to pull you through the rougher moments and days.

5. Explore complementary medicine treatments for dealing with side effects, such as calendula-based creams, massage and acupuncture (see Chapter 12).

6. Hang in there. You are nearing the end of treatment.

[18]

Transitioning Forward

Update #19 - March 6

One of the issues that I have been struggling with as I near the end of treatment is how to resume my life. Do I slip back into the way things were before all this started or do I live life as if each day is a precious gift, an unexpected bonus that should be milked for all its worth? I guess my tentative answer is somewhere in the middle. My life before cancer was a pretty wonderful one. While cancer is some kind of wake-up call – or knock on the head – I felt that I was alive, with my eyes wide open, savoring the good times, aware of a range of feelings, living the "examined life." On the other hand, this has certainly given me an opportunity to fine tune, to decide what is extraneous and can be tossed, what I would like to modify, and where I want to put my energies. No conclusions yet, just a lot of thoughts.

I t looks easy. It should be easy.

Treatments were finished. No more chemo. There were some residual side effects, but no new ones. No more daily treks to radiation. No more surgery in the offing.

Hurray! This was certainly a time for celebration, and celebrate I did.

The last few weeks of radiation were filled with the grateful anticipation of what was to come. I spent my time and energies planning my celebratory vacations, trying to focus on them and forget the dreary waiting room in the dungeon of the radiotherapy department. In contrast to the feelings I had when I finished chemo, when I had the strong desire to celebrate with family, community and friends, this time I wanted none of that. I wanted to fly the coop and get as far away as I could. I was free! No need to be near hospitals, doctors, or anything to do with cancer.

I planned my escape carefully: a five-day stay at a health farm up north followed by a nine-day trip to Venice. I have always noticed that the anticipation of vacation is equally valuable and sometimes more enjoyable than the vacation itself. This time around, not only did I thoroughly enjoy the planning and picturing myself in these exotic locations, they actually carried me through some of my rougher moments towards the end of radiation treatment, when my patience ran extremely thin. But anticipations aside, the vacations were absolutely wonderful. The time at the detox farm was healing for my body. We spent the days walking (naturally, since this vacation was spent with my reliable walking partner), doing Qi Gong (a gentle form of Chinese exercise), yoga, massages, eating very healthy meals and listening to lectures about nutrition and health.

The vacation in Venice was magical, as is the city of Venice itself. Our apartment, located on one of the major waterways, allowed me to spend long hours just watching the busy boat traffic stream by on the murky waters surrounding the island.

As the days at the health farm were healing for my body, so the days in Venice were balm for my soul. On the evening of the third day of our enchanted stay in Venice, I remarked to my husband that I hadn't thought about cancer once the entire day. I couldn't believe it! Hopefully, this was a taste of what was to come.

After nine days filled with sights, sounds, a good combination of relaxation and activity, it was time to come back to life. Real life. I was transitioning once again, in this year filled with transitions. This time, however, I thought it would be a piece of cake. I thought I would be resuming a life with which I was familiar. I would be picking up the pieces of my life before cancer. But as I continue to learn, life isn't always what you expect.

Upon returning from vacation, I found that there was a strong subliminal message surrounding me that went something like this: "Phew! It's over! That's wonderful! Now we can put this cancer behind us. You are just like us now." Yet, I found myself hesitating to jump right into the celebration. I wasn't ready yet. I kept thinking to myself, "Am I really over it? Am I really just like them (those healthy folks)?" And then, "I am not there yet. I am still IN it. Don't you understand?" Meanwhile, I wondered to myself, "What is the big rush? Is it really so hard for the people around me to think about cancer, or about ME having cancer?" I know that cancer comes along with a host of issues that are often less than pleasant to deal with, for example: mortality, suffering, death, fears and anxieties. I know that my friends and family were truly happy for me that I had completed cancer treatments and was still in one piece, but I wanted to say to them, "Slow down, I am not finished yet. I am still dealing with cancer and its aftermath every single day."

Was I like the holocaust survivor who had stories nobody wanted to hear? Or the soldier who has returned from battle, whose grateful family does all they can in order not to hear his gruesome battle stories? Was it society that was shutting me up? Or was I misreading the situation? I was sure that nobody could quite understand what I had been through, and if they did, they wouldn't know what to do with it anyway. While I knew that I was reasonably intact, I felt that my re-entry into the world was reminiscent of many trauma survivors whose stories have gone unheard and unsung.

After getting all worked up about how I seemed to be out of sync with the world around me, I began to wonder to myself whether I had become spoiled and perhaps was having a hard time giving up cancer because somehow it made me special. Had I gotten used to being the center of attention, to all the special treatment that goes along with having cancer, and actually liked it? I recalled what I had learned way back in grad school about the secondary gains that sick people often enjoy. These can include social, financial, or personal gains that may encourage them to stay in their patient role, far beyond the limits dictated by their disease. I knew for sure I didn't want to be a cancer patient, yet there were elements of this time period that were very sweet. For example, my husband's tender affection and his willingness to do it MY way, all the time, without discussion. Or, my kids' extra attention and alacrity in putting everything aside to come and spend time with me was wonderful. The palpable feeling of love and caring surrounding me and the living of each day with a mindfulness that added both depth and purpose were all part of the sweetness of life that cancer had brought. I was going to miss all of that. Did I have to give it all up so quickly? Did I have to give it up at all?

In addition to the attention, love and kindness showered upon me, there had been the more material benefits that came along with having cancer. These included the income tax break, and the extra insurance income, as well as the time off from work and the handicapped parking sticker, which allowed me to park more easily wherever I went. I would surely miss those perks.

Yet above and beyond what I have listed here, there was the more subtle feeling that I was somehow special during this year of cancer. I was going through something different than the people around me, something that clearly marked me off as unique, a little beyond the pale. I savored that feeling, as I have always enjoyed being a little bit off the main track. I like to think my own thoughts, do my own thing, and go my own way. I have always disliked crowds and shied away from the herd mentality. This cancer thing had clearly set me apart and made me different in a very external and obvious way. The suffering that goes along with cancer is not only private and intimate, it generally has a pretty public aspect, too. When you go bald, everyone knows you are undergoing chemo. When the word gets out, people are very kind and solicitous, constantly asking you how you are feeling

This is in contrast to the experience of those who suffer a variety of other physical diseases, mental illnesses, family problems or financial woes, all of whom may live with their distress silently. Often, nobody around them knows what they are going through. Typically, nobody pays attention. Seldom do people ask how they feel or offer support until the situation gets so desperate that it can no longer be overlooked.

Cancer is different. When you have cancer, and you choose to live it publicly, the outpouring is immense. For some reason, cancer hits a nerve in most people. I often wonder whether they think, "Whew! Glad it's her and not me!" Or perhaps they think something more along the lines of, "If it happened to her, it could happen to me too!" Or does cancer push all of us to the cliff's edge, forcing us to look over and to realize that we are all going to die some day? I am not sure exactly what the mechanism is, but whatever it is, the interest, the questions, the feeling of support, and even admiration for how I had "handled it", had been immense. How could I give that up and go back to being a regular person, living a regular life?

Several weeks before I completed treatment my brother, who had survived a bout with cancer himself some twenty-five years earlier, told me that he had some advice for me about "life after cancer." I eagerly set a date with him for lunch so that we could have some serious conversation, unlike the kind you have at family events. After a glass of wine, some appetizers and introductory chit chat our conversation took a serious turn. He talked about his feelings when he completed treatment. His bottom line for me was that, in his experience, the force of life is so strong that it will sweep you away and take over, sending you right back into the maelstrom, unless you keep up your guard. For my brother, it was very easy to just pick up the pieces where he had left off and abandon all his newfound wisdom within a few weeks. Gone were the resolutions about changing priorities and living his life differently. Life had taken over.

My brother's wisdom reverberated inside of me. I felt that pull. It would be so easy to go back to life pre-cancer. Aside from the background noise of dark thoughts and worries, and an aching underarm, everything could be the same as it had been. Is that what I wanted? Life was good before cancer: I had a good job, a great family, a nice home in a community I had chosen. What was wrong with going back to all that? I lived the considered life before cancer. I breathed. I meditated. I was mindful. I exercised. I ate healthfully. I had an exciting career and a rich spiritual life. It sounds good. It was good. But I was different now. For the last ten months I had lived every day recognizing that it was a gift, not to be taken lightly or for granted. That recognition was something that I wanted to keep in   my forebrain, ever present, always with me, forever. How was I to do that?

When I was initially diagnosed with cancer and death reared its head, it became a very present reality in my life. At that point I did not know the extent of my cancer, and whether it had spread. I began to review my life, examining what I had accomplished and all the things I had not yet done but were still waiting for me. The proverbial "bucket list." It was not an easy task for me to make that list. My powers of planning and projection beyond the span of a few weeks have never been very well developed. I tend to take things as they come. I now recognize and respect that my inability to plan long-term stems not from a deficit but rather from the humble awareness that my ability to control the future is limited, and from the desire to take full advantage of what life sends me in the here and now.

So how was I to create a "bucket list" now and what might be on it? Travel, travel and more travel. But not just any travel. I realized that when I travel I want to meet real people, and get to know the country, culture, and places to which I travel. Moving beyond the narrow horizons that cancer treatment had shoved upon me, I was eager to set off. I had been fortunate over the last few years to have the opportunity to visit many places in the world, in order to teach people about trauma and building resilience, and I enjoyed these encounters immensely. So the idea of travel combined with work was high on my list. Writing a book was on the list, as I had always enjoyed writing, and felt that by writing I could explore familiar terrain and perhaps dig deeper, find out more, and share some of my wisdom with interested readers. Other things on my list were spending more time with my grandchildren and my aging parents. That's about it.

What did I need to rearrange in order to help make that list a reality? I thought long and hard and decided to cut back at work, from a 100% full-time position to working only three days a week. During my year of cancer I had definitely enjoyed not being a slave to work. The decision to cut back officially was not too difficult, primarily because of the wonderful team with whom I worked. By working only three days a week, I had an additional three days "off". These free days have given me the opportunity to pursue writing, spend more time with family and continue to focus on the healing that I still need to do. This change in my life has also allowed me the luxury of time, which I can dedicate to being mindful about my priorities. Rearranging my weekly schedule has encouraged me not to slip too readily back into old, pre-cancer patterns.

One of the great lessons I learned from cancer is not to put things off, but rather to take advantage of the time I have right now. I often remind myself that time is an illusion, and even though I am feeling wonderful today, it can change at the drop of a hat. If I have an opportunity now, I grab it with both hands.

In the last three months I have written a book, couch surfed and cycled the Netherlands with my daughter, and spent a lot of time with the grandkids. And I am looking forward to further adventures. Today, as I write the conclusion of this book, I am taking my parents for a ride to see the spring flowers, and am packing for a one-week trip to Indonesia, to teach about trauma and building resilience in the face of disaster. For this I am grateful.

Update #20 - April 19

I am giving notice:

This is my final update, at least for now. I think this is habit forming, and it is time to move on. This is another way of saying that I am going through yet another transition on this winding, healing journey. As most of you know, I finished radiation treatment about two months ago. As planned, I spent a fabulous month vacationing and celebrating my newfound freedom.

I find it remarkable that my cancer journey was mirrored by the seasons. I was diagnosed in June, had surgery in July, began chemo in August and completed it in late November. During that time we had the mourning period for the destruction of the Temple in Jerusalem more than 2,000 years ago (culminating in the 9th of Av), the High Holy Days which afforded me the chance to do a very serious examining of my soul, my life, and my priorities, and then we moved into the very short dark days of the year, just as the chemo was at its peak. I had further surgery in January, followed by radiation. As radiation wore on, the days got longer, my hope got stronger, and spring sprung. I could actually see the moment that spring arrived as our train pulled into Venice. When we arrived at the train station, at the outskirts of the city, the last few raindrops of winter fell, and the clouds in the sky began to lift. After setting out from the station, as our waterbus navigated the canals, we saw the setting sun peek out between the clouds. We had eight glorious sun- filled days of spring weather there, followed by an amazingly green and flower-filled spring back home. It is amazing to me how nature and the cycle of the year mirrored my personal journey. Now, once again, I feel like I am transitioning and, in a way being born again - back into "regular life", thank God.

I am picking up this email update about two weeks later, and this time I am determined to finish and get this off. Yesterday I finished my second "checkup", and got signed off by the surgeon. A few weeks ago I was signed off by the oncologist. They both want to see me occasionally (the oncologist more often, the surgeon less often), and I will be doing a mammography once a year (I hope), and a breast MRI once a year. That is the extent of the tests and follow-up at this point. It does sound hopeful. When I said goodbye to the surgeon yesterday he said, "See you in a year, God willing." That's what this is all about: God willing. I think cancer has given me some humility in that corner, reminding me that what I think is in my hands, really isn't. It's just an illusion.

So that's it folks. Thanks for hearing me out all these long months, and for all the wonderful e-mails you have sent in return. I loved each and every one of them. Your support and love have meant the world to me. I treasure them.

Love,

Naomi

TIPS ON TRANSITIONING BACK INTO LIFE:

1. Go slow. Even though the rest of the world thinks that you have completed cancer treatment and can put it behind you, you know that it takes time.

2. Figure out your priorities for the next few months and make a list. Don't wait too long to make the "perfect" list, because life will take over and carry you away.

3. Revisit and revise your list at regular intervals, checking to see how you are doing, and what else has come up. Remember that life is
dynamic and all the planning in the world only goes so far.

The journey continues to unfold and I am an eager traveler. Thanks for coming along for the ride.

Appendix I: How to Build Resilience:
My Professional Journey

I went into the field of psychology to help people. I also like to hear life stories, and I thought this would give me a window into lives other than my own, as I tried to help them. After having been a school psychologist for more than twenty years, I was ready to explore new fields and gain new expertise, and so I transitioned into the world of trauma psychology. My decision to focus on trauma and resilience building grew out of the pressing geo-political situation of the Second Intifada (Palestinian uprising in the years 2000-2005), which increasingly brought the threat of terror attack, and actual loss of limb and life, very close to home.

At the time the Second Intifada broke out in September, 2001, I was a Fellow at the Mandel School for Educational Leadership. This was the first time in more than twenty years that I was taking a hiatus from professional life, and enjoying the freedom of scholarly study in the fields of philosophy, education and policy-making. I was having a ball, thoroughly enjoying myself as I immersed myself in the study of texts, writing papers, and endless discussions with other Fellows. The responsibilities of the day-to-day running of the Psychological Services Unit in the municipal region of Gush

Etzion was fading from my consciousness. Children with learning problems or emotional problems, frazzled teachers and parents, were all becoming a thing of the past. Then the Intifada started, with suicide bombers blowing themselves up on buses, in coffee shops, and any place there was a crowd, throughout Jerusalem. The road from my home in Gush Etzion to Jerusalem became a sniper-infested route, and as we could not afford to bulletproof our cars, we took to wearing bulletproof vests and helmets for the fifteen-minute drive to Jerusalem every day. This was a scary time indeed. My thoughts and heart went out to my colleagues from whom I had so recently parted at the Psychological Services Unit of Gush Etzion. I wanted to be there to help them and the community during this trying time. I talked about my dilemma at length with the director of the Mandel School of Educational Leadership, a very sharp and creative woman. She urged me to take both my knowledge, the time and resources afforded to me by the Mandel School, along with my driving motivation of wanting to help the communities closest to me both in Gush Etzion and Jerusalem, and see what I could create.

That conversation was the impetus for the "Building Resilience Intervention" (BRI), which became my personal project while at Mandel, and eventually the basis of my work for the next decade at the Israel Center for the Treatment of Psychotrauma. What I laid out in the BRI was a model of intervention in communities and schools whose members had been exposed to trauma, natural disaster, or the threat of trauma. After spending a lot of time reading the psychological literature, and talking with people in government, academia, and other institutions, I came to the conclusion that, while there was a fairly well-established and mapped out immediate response to trauma, there were no programs that dealt with the long-term or ongoing effects of trauma or disaster. Just as the debris and detritus from terror attacks were cleaned up with remarkable alacrity and efficiency, so too the mental health response was both efficient and quick. But what happened one week later? One month later? One year later? How were teachers and parents coping? What was happening to the kids? This is what concerned me and this became my focus.

The BRI model that I developed and subsequently implemented with thousands of teachers, all over Israel and in far-flung places such as Mexico, the Gulf Coast of Mississippi, and Haiti, posits that there are four cornerstones or pillars of resilience. These four cornerstones that I termed the four S's include:

1. Self
2. Strengths
3. Support
4. Significance

Now let me explain what I mean by each one of these "pillars". Self is the first one. It lays the foundation for all subsequent work. Self refers to the understanding that body and soul are strongly connected. Stress affects both body and soul, as does trauma, crisis and disaster. There are skills and practices that one can learn to reduce the stress response in the body and to return to a greater sense of equilibrium. The unit on Self includes quite a bit of psycho-education about stress and trauma, as well as teaching breathing, meditation and guided imagery. In this unit workshop participants have a chance to explore how the trauma, stress or crisis is affecting them personally as well as how they are impacted in their professional lives.

An anecdote is in order here to illustrate this point. I arrived in Biloxi, Mississippi, together with a co-worker, in November 2006. Fifteen months after Hurricane Katrina had pounded this coastal town wreaking havoc in its wake. We asked the teachers we were working with to draw pictures of where they were a week after the hurricane and where they were now. The purpose of this exercise was to give the teachers a quiet time to reflect on the changes in their lives since the hurricane, without revisiting the most traumatic moments of the hurricane itself. The teachers enthusiastically threw themselves into the task and began to draw. When they completed drawing, as we went around the circle and they shared their drawings, many of them had tears in their eyes. They said that this was the first time since the hurricane that they had stopped to reflect about themselves and their feelings. They related that they had each been so frantically busy helping others – students, family members, and friends – that they had not taken the time to check in with themselves and see how they were doing. The unit on Self encourages participants to have a look inside, to check in and see what's up. How am I doing? How am I feeling? What is happening with me?

The second pillar of the BRI, Strengths, refers to the internal strength to express emotion. In this unit, we unpack some of the emotions that run rampant during times of trauma and crisis including, but not limited to, fear, anxiety, shock, sadness, grief, and loss. In this unit we have opportunities to do creative work using non-verbal avenues such as sculpting or making collages to express these emotions. After allowing non-verbal expression, we move into translating these feelings into words.

This is a necessary step if we are to speak with our children, students and people around us about difficult emotions. People are often afraid to talk about difficult things, but I have always been drawn to just that—talking about difficult things. I now know that this is an essential skill if we are to bridge the gap between folks, reach out to those in need and create a feeling of community and support. There is nothing like silence to create a sense of isolation, a feeling that no one can understand you and that you, indeed, are all alone. All these feelings can merely exacerbate an already bad situation. Teaching empathic communication opens doors. Communication brings down barriers between people and creates a road to healing.

The third pillar of the BRI, Social Supports, actually represents the foremost resource that helps people cope during times of trouble. In this unit we focus on the existing coping patterns people have, explore ways of expanding these resources and trying out new behaviors, activities, or skills. We also have a look at the social supports available to us, and examine how and why we make use of them the way we do.

The final pillar of the BRI is Significance, and this relates to finding meaning and hope in one's experiences. In the psychological literature Viktor Frankl is the grandfather of logotherapy, and of most fields of psychology related to meaning. He says in many different ways that if you have a "what" to live for, you can endure most anything, and he should know. He was a Holocaust survivor who endured long months and years in the Nazi concentration camp, Auschwitz, hanging on to his life by a thread because of the "what" that he had to live for. In our intervention, we allow a place to ask questions and to consider the meaning of the difficult things that happen to us, without having to arrive at a "final" or "correct" answer.

The search for meaning in difficult situations is a naturally occurring behavior after trauma or tragedy. Many quash this most human of pursuits because they feel that it gets them nowhere or that they don't have the answers. We have found that when we make a space for this exploration without promising answers, it can be a most empowering and enriching exercise. Not only adults, but children too, are often trying to figure out why these bad things are happening to them and what they can do about it. Assuring parents and teachers that they don't have to have all the answers encourages them to open this topic up with children of all ages as well.

Accompanying these pillars of the BRI are manuals and workbooks that we have developed to aid workshop participants in carrying this healing method back into their own personal and professional lives. In the manuals and workbooks there are exercises related to each one of these topics. For example, in the section on Self there is a script for guided imagery to a safe place. (The guided imagery script is included in the index of this book.) There is also a work sheet called "Stress Mapping," in which the user is asked to list and map out current stresses in his or her life. In the section on Significance there is an exercise for younger students in which they are asked to interview parents or grandparents about overcoming a difficult experience in their lives whether it is war, poverty, disability, discrimination or other personal crisis.

Now that I have given a rather lengthy description of my professional work, how does all of this impact on who I am and what happens to me when I meet my own personal trauma? Discovering that you have cancer is traumatic indeed. It fits all the criteria for trauma:

It happens suddenly (for most people and certainly for me)

It is life threatening

It is usually accompanied by strong feelings of fear and helplessness and a sense of loss of control

To backtrack for a moment – exactly what is trauma? Several years ago, I wrote that the original meaning of the Greek word "trauma" is wound, or damage to body tissue. Today we use the term "psychological trauma" to describe a condition in which a person has experienced a difficult event that has wounded his or her psyche. The traumatic event is usually unpredictable and uncontrollable. It may shatter our sense of security and leave us feeling vulnerable and agitated. The event does not have to be one in which the person is directly involved. Sometimes the news of the death of someone close to us can be traumatic. People who watch traumatic news events on television may report feeling traumatized as well.

So, I experienced a trauma, and it was both physical and psychological. Did all my training and background help me? I think so. How? Firstly, I was able to mobilize resources that often help people in trauma. I was able to recognize that the distress I was feeling in my most uncomfortable moments was probably normal. Within days I began regularly practicing guided imagery to help me calm down, feel more regulated and in control. I was able to talk freely about my feelings, my fears, and my distress, sometimes ad nauseum I am sure, but thankfully I had a good listener in my husband Mike and some of my good friends. I was able to share relatively easily with my children, extended family and colleagues, which brought an outpouring of support, love and caring. I was confident enough to assertively ask my doctors for more information when I didn't understand, or needed to have something repeated or needed to find out more. I actively pursued complementary forms of healing. All this came from my experiences in resilience building, and the knowledge that the active, engaged pursuit of healing was probably the best antidote to feelings of helplessness and despair.

So the short answer is yes. Being a professional in the resilience building and trauma field definitely came to my aid at this time. My oncologist often joked with me about how resilient I had to be because I was the "Director of the Resilience Unit", but in fact it was true. Resilience was in my very being, my blood, my DNA, who I am. When explaining what resilience building is all about, I often say that when we talk about resilience we are coming from a perspective of looking at the cup that is half full. By that I mean that we ask questions like: What resources do you have? What strengths do you have? And we build on those. This is in contrast to clinical psychology that often looks at the cup that is half empty and focuses on what is wrong with you, asking questions like: What are you missing? What is pathological? What do we need to fix? The resilience approach is very empowering. It posits a basic faith in human nature. It rests upon a trust that when given the right environment of support and caring, people will be able to find the right road for themselves. Having been steeped in this optimistic tradition for a decade or more before being diagnosed with cancer, I was primed and ready to take the cancer head on.

Appendix II:
Professional Articles
by Naomi L. Baum

Baum, N. L., Stokar, Y. N., Ginat, R., Ziv, Y., Abu-Jufar, I., Cardozo, B. L., Pat-Horenczyk, R., & Brom, D. (in press). Building resilience intervention (BRI) with teachers in Bedouin communities: From evidence informed to evidence based. *The International Journal of Education*.

Brom, D., **Baum, N.L.**, & Pat-Horenczyk , R. (in press) Systems of care for traumatized children: The example of a School-based Intervention model. In: H.S. Wallach, M.P. Safir & A. Rizzo (Eds.) **Future Directions in PTSD: Diagnosis, Prevention, and Treatment**. New York: Springer

Stokar, Y. N., **Baum, N. L.**, Plischke, A., & Ziv, Y. (2014). The key to resilience: A peer based youth leader training and support program. **Journal of Child and Adolescent Trauma.**

Baum, N. L., Ginat, R., & Silverman, P. R. (2014). Childhood bereavement and traumatic loss. In Pat-Horenczyk, R., Brom, D., Chemtob, C., & Vogel, J. (Eds.), **Helping children cope with trauma: Individual family and community perspectives.** Routledge.

Baum, N. L., Brom, D., Pat-Horenczyk, Rahabi, S., Wardi, J. & Weltman, A. (2013). Transitioning from the battlefield to home: An innovative program for Israeli soldiers. **Journal of Aggression, Maltreatment & Trauma**, 22(6), 644-659.

Baum, N. L., Lopes-Cardozo, B., Pat-Horenczyk, R., Ziv, Y., Blanton, C., Reza, A., Weltman, A., & Brom, D. (2013). Training teachers to build resilience in children in the aftermath of war: A cluster randomized trial. **Child & Youth Care Forum**. 42, 339-350.

Astor, R. A., Benbenishty, R., Pat-Horenczyk, R., Brom, D., **Baum, N.,** Schiff, M., & De Pedro, K. (2012). The Influence of the Second Lebanese War on Israeli Students in Urban School Settings: Findings of the Nahariya District-Wide Screening Prototype. In: Gallagher, K.S., Brewer, D., Goodyear, R., Bensimon., E., & Picus, L. (Eds.) **International handbook of research in urban education**. New York: Taylor & Francis.

Schiff, M., Pat-Horenczyk, R., Benbenishty, R., Brom, D., **Baum, N**., & Astor, R.A. (2012). High school students' posttraumatic symptoms, substance abuse and involvement in violence in the aftermath of war. **Social Science & Medicine,** 75, 1321-1328.

Brom, D., Pat-Horenczyk, R. & **Baum, N.L.** (2011). The influence of war and terrorism on post traumatic distress among Israeli children. **International Psychiatry**, 8 (4), 81-83.

Pat-Horenczyk, R., Brom, D., **Baum. N.**, Benbenishty, R., Schiff, M. & Astor, R. A. (2011). A city-wide school-based model for addressing the needs of children exposed to terrorism and war. In: V. Ardino (Ed.) **Post-traumatic syndromes in children and adolescents.** Wiley/Blackwell Press.

Schiff, M., Pat-Horenczyk, R., Benbenishty, R., Brom, D., **Baum, N.**, & Astor, R.A. (2010). Seeking help: Do adolescents know when they need help? Jewish and Arab youths report on their posttraumatic distress in the aftermath of war. **Journal of Traumatic Stress,** 23(5), 657-660.

Baum, N.L., Reidler, E., Rotter, B., & Brom, D. (2009). Building resilience in schools in the wake of Hurricane Katrina. **Journal of Child and Adolescent Trauma,** 2(1).

Baum, N.L., Rotter, B., & Reidler, E. (2009) Building resilience for holocaust educators. **Prism**, 1(1), 81-88.

Baum, N. L. & Rotter, B. (2008). **"My Resilience Workbook."** Israel Center for the Treatment of Psychotrauma, Jerusalem, Israel. In house published workbook for children to cope with trauma. Over 5,000 distributed.

Brody, D. and **Baum, N.L.** (2007). Israel kindergarten teachers cope with terror and war: Two implicit models of resilience. **Curriculum Inquiry,** 37. 9-33.

Baum, Naomi L. (2005). Building resilience in the preschool classroom: A psychoeducational response to expsure to terror. In E. Somer and A. Bleich (Eds) **Israel Responds to Terrorism**. Tel Aviv: Ramot (published in Hebrew).

Baum, N.L. (2004) Building Resilience: A School Based Intervention for Children Exposed to ongoing Trauma and

Stress. In Y. Danieli, D. Brom, and J. Sills (Eds.) **The Trauma of Terrorism: An International handbook of Shared Knowledge and Shared Care**. Haworth Press.

Baum, N.L., Bamberger, E., & Kerem, R. (2004). **Building resilience in the classroom: Teacher's manual.** Self published manual, Israel Center for the Treatment of Psychotrauma, Jerusalem, Israel.

Baum, N.L..& Kerem, R. (2004). **Building resilience**: A **facilitator's guide.** Self published manual, Israel Center for the Treatment of Psychotrauma, Jerusalem, Israel.

Baum, N.L., Bamberger, E.. & Anchor, C. (2004). **Building resilience in the preschool: Teacher's manual.** Self published manual, Israel Center for the Treatment of Psychotrauma, Jerusalem, Israel.

Baum, Naomi L. (1996). Educating towards prayer -- a qualitative research experience. **Derekh Efrata** -- Journal of Efrata Teachers' College.

Baum, Naomi L. Kravitz, S., Katz, S. (1981). Relationships between age, social activity, meaningful activity and life satisfaction. **Bitahon sociale**, Journal of the Israel Association of Social Workers, 22, 71-76.

Loewenberg, Naomi (1976). Coping with death. **Harefuah**, Journal of the Israel Medical Association, 91, 39-42.

Acknowledgements

It is a singular pleasure to reach the end of this book and thank all of those people who have been there for me, first during my year of cancer, and then during the adventure of writing this book.

First thanks goes to my family: to Mike - my life's partner, our children and grandchildren, our parents, brothers and sisters (in-laws as well) who never wavered, were there to support, to cheer me on, to laugh with me and distract me, to cry with me, morning, noon and night. You pulled me through.

A special thank you to my editor and friend Channah Koppel for her good cheer, insightful questions and good counsel. Noga Fisher my walking partner was there with me when the seed for this book germinated, and walked me through many a rough moment and for that I am grateful. Heartfelt thanks to Deborah Harris, whose friendship I found through cancer, and who advised, read and encouraged me through this book, so that I could be a voice not only for me, but also for her and for many other fellow travelers on this breast cancer path as well.

I am grateful to Ricardo Lowenberg, artist and long lost cousin who graciously allowed me to use his amazing painting, "Tree of Life", for my cover. Ricardo's works can be found at: www.ricardolowenberg.com.

To my colleagues from the Israel Center for the Treatment of Psychotrauma who have been such wonderful friends for the last twelve years and during my year of healing from cancer held my hand, supported me in every way possible, cheered me on, cooked for me and much much more.

To my fantastic medical team: Dr. Karen Djamal, my family physician and dear friend, Dr. Moshe Carmon, breast surgeon par excellence, and Dr. Amiel Segal, the straightest shooter that ever walked this earth, I say thank you from the bottom of my heart. To Dr. Gechtman, my "angel" who found the small node in my underarm and allowed the healing to begin, words are not enough to express my heartfelt gratitude.

And finally last but certainly not least, to my dear friends across the years and over the oceans, in Israel and abroad, who stayed in touch, prayed for me, hoped with me, read my e-mails and answered them, rooted for me, and made me feel ever so loved. Thank you all.

In conclusion, I end with the words of the Psalm 55:23 that have accompanied me on this long and sometimes arduous path, "Cast your cares on the Lord, and He will sustain you," for in the end it is all in God's hands and there I rest.

Picture Album

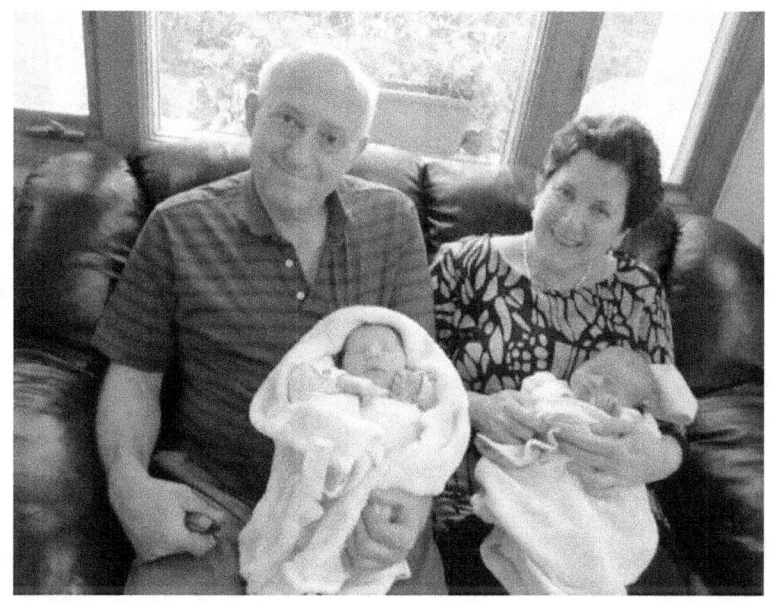

March, 2011 -- Before Diagnosis with our newest grandchildren

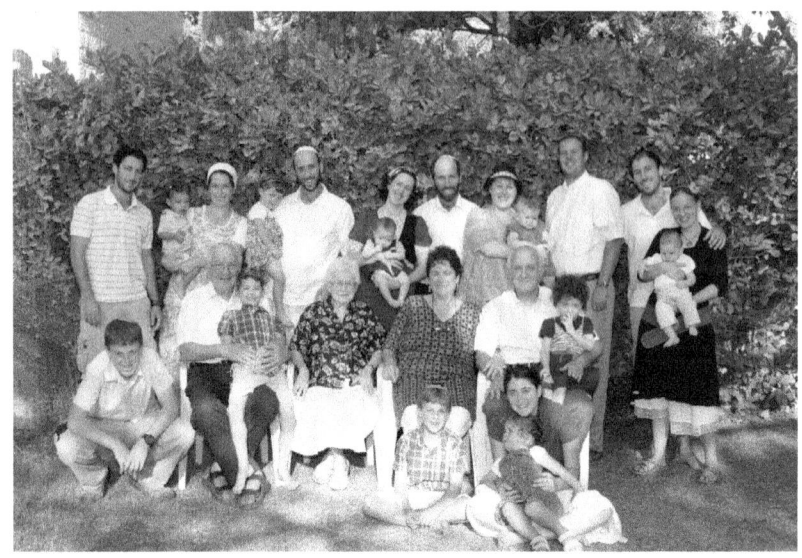

The entire clan - July, 2011 -two days after diagnosis

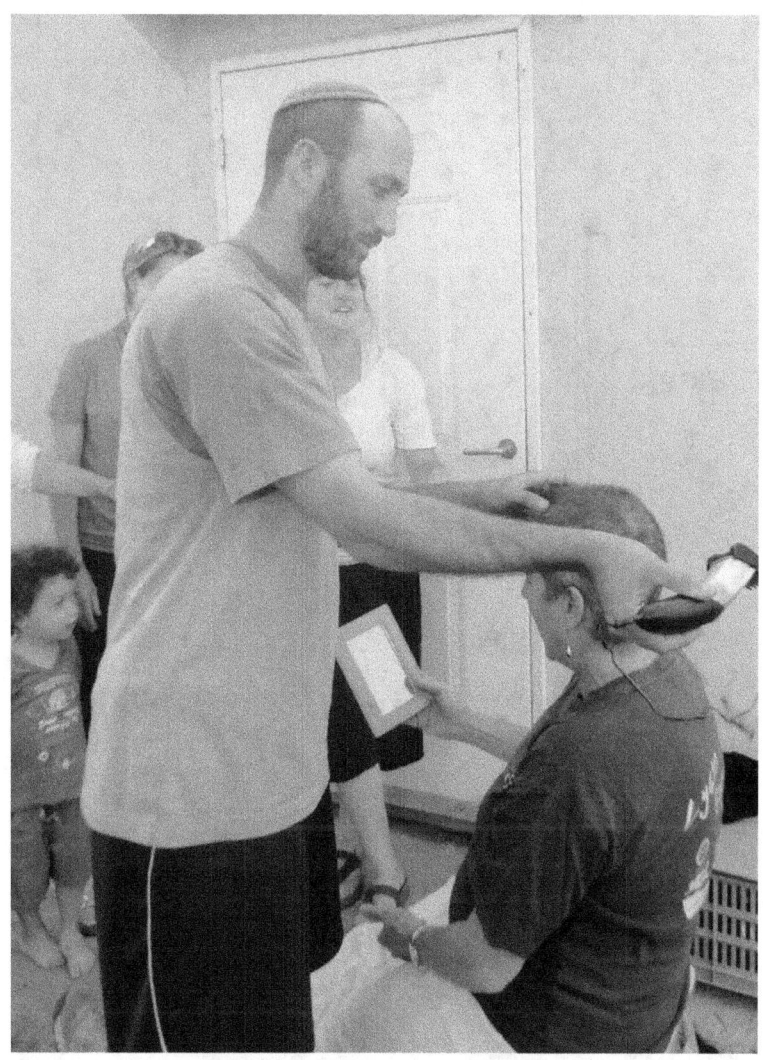

Home Haircut- Eitan is the Barber

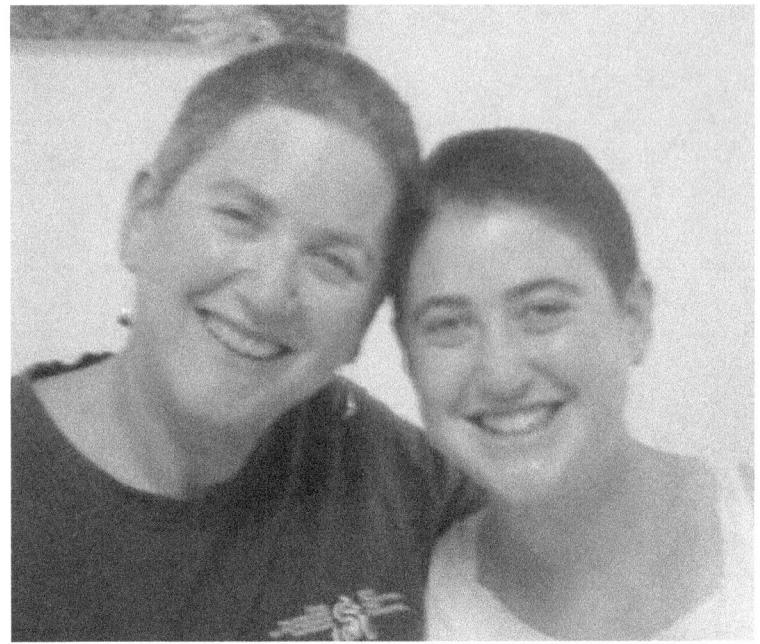

Shlomzion and Me - Twin Haircuts

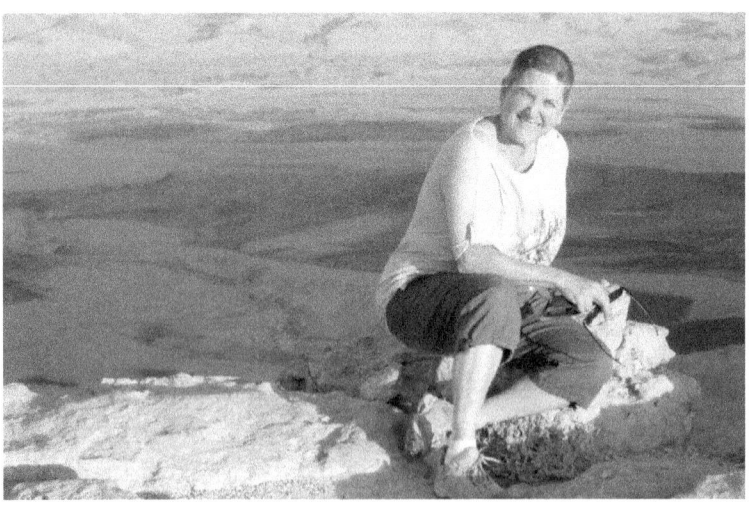

Vacation after first round of chemo - Mizpeh Ramon

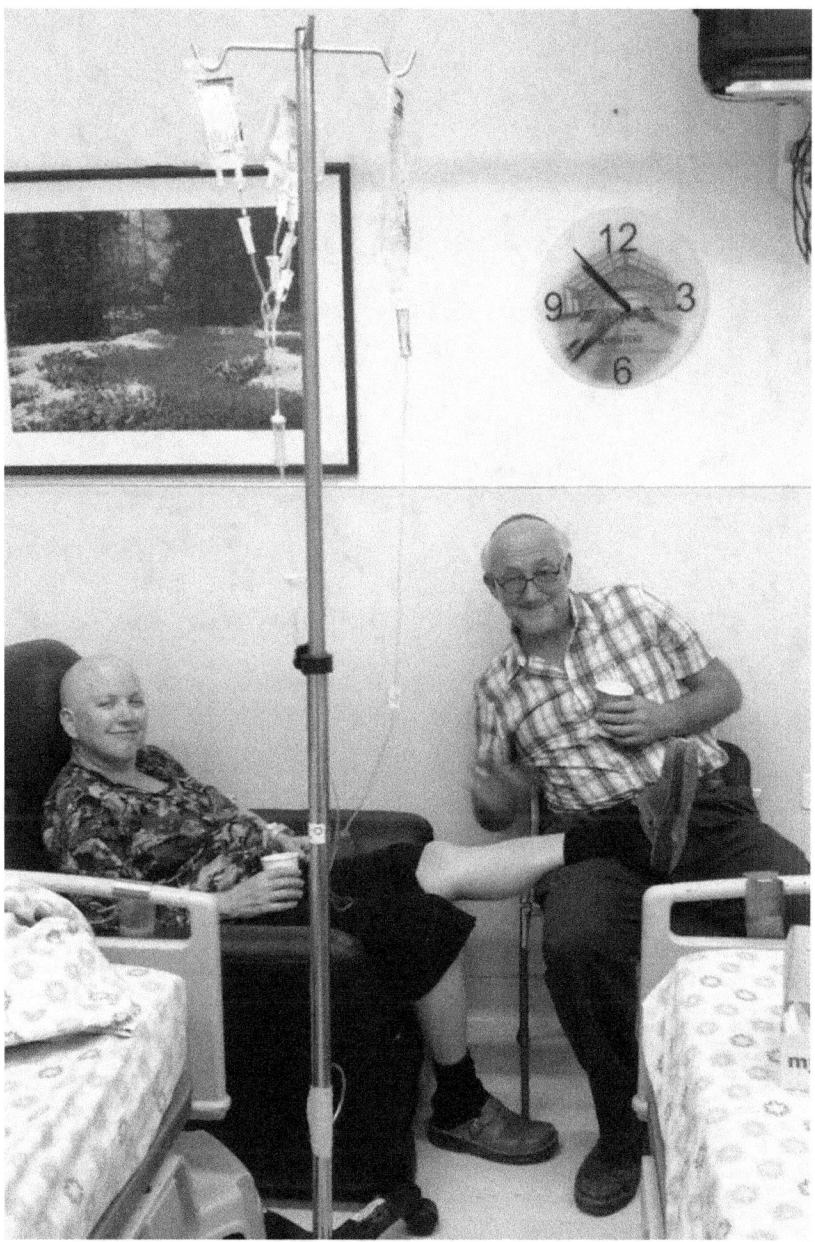

Last chemo session with Mike

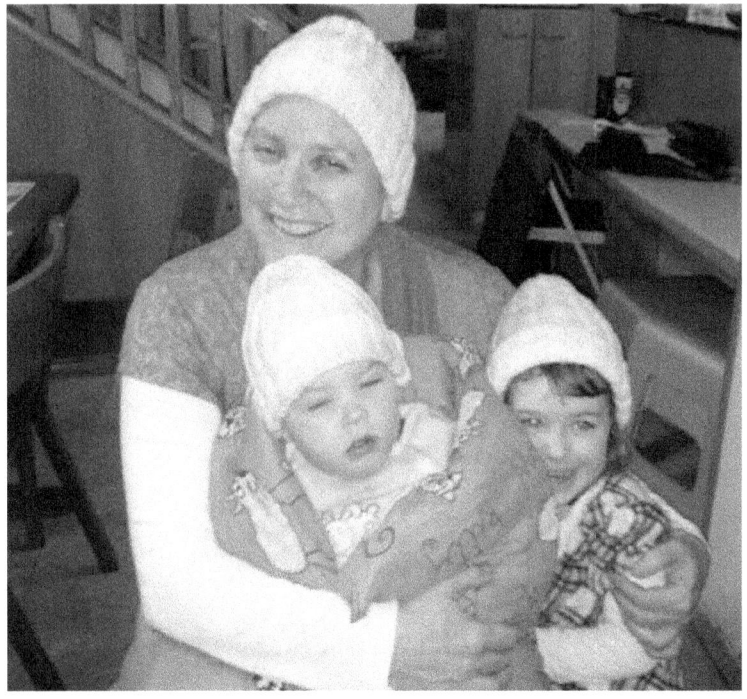

Wearing matching hats made by Grandma

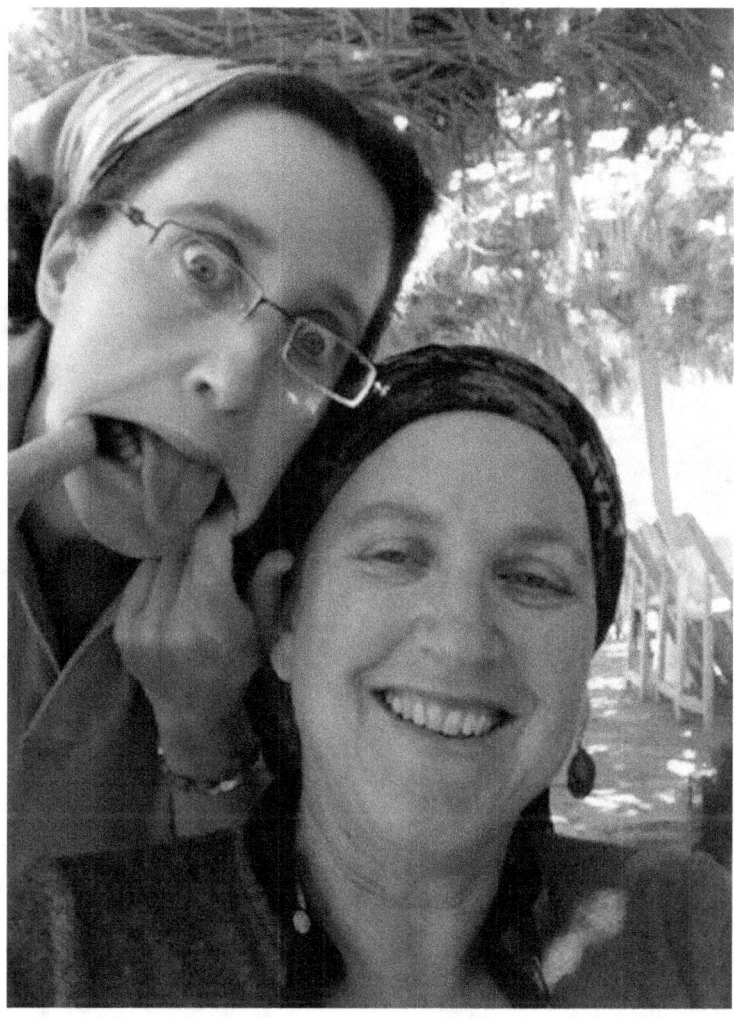

The "scarf look" with Shoshi

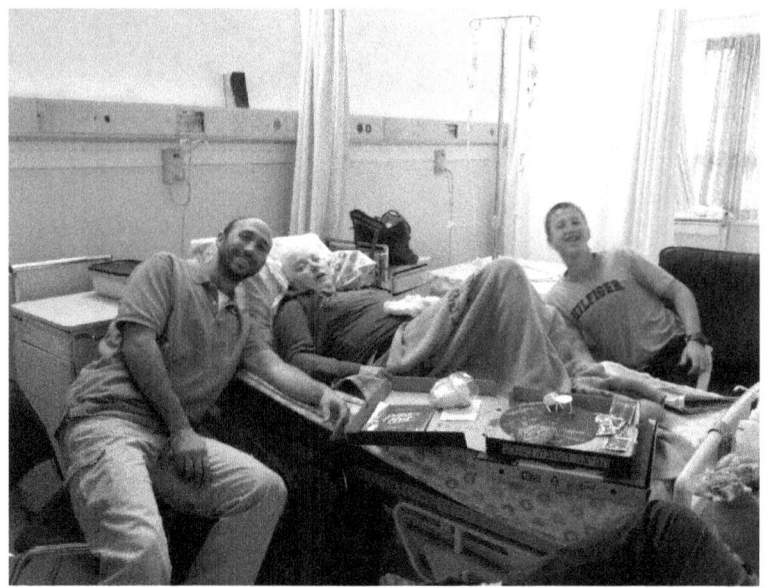

Pizza party at last chemo - with Eitan and Neriya

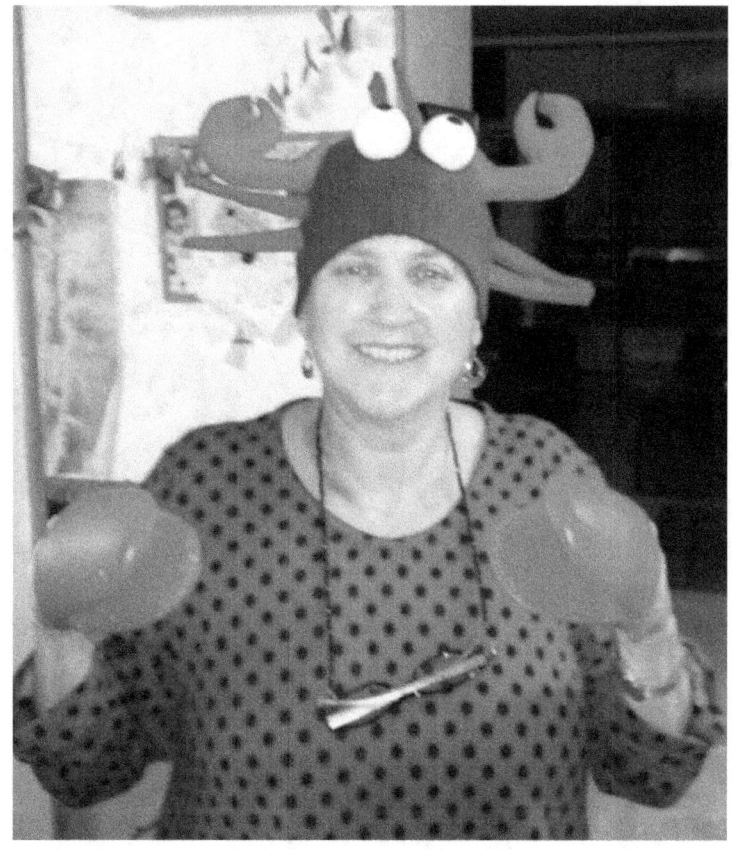

Purim costume on last day of radiation- dressed up as a "cancer" crab

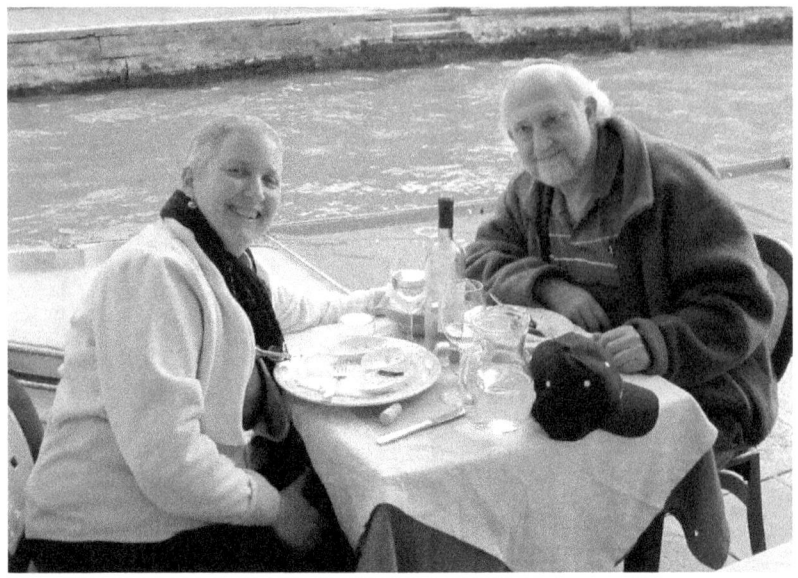

Celebrating life in Venice - April, 2012

About the Author

Naomi Baum is a psychologist and Director of the Resilience Unit at the Israel Center for the Treatment of Psychotrauma, in Jerusalem as well as Senior Consulting Psychologist from Chai Lifeline-Project Chai in New York. She received her Ph.D. from Bryn Mawr College in the USA. She has been a consulting psychologist for schools, and taught courses in psychology at the university level in both the USA and Israel. She has created and implemented resilience-building programs for those exposed to trauma. In addition to working extensively with schools and parents she has applied her model of resilience building to work with first responders, rabbis, nurses, and many other communities affected by trauma. This work has taken her to such far-flung places as Haiti, Mexico and Biloxi, Mississippi. While Naomi has accrued many degrees and much work experience, her real understanding of kids and families comes from being married to the same man for almost forty years, and raising, with him, their seven children. She is the proud grandmother of twelve. Her hobbies include scuba diving, travelling, reading and biking. She lives with her husband in Efrat, Israel.

She can be reached at www.naomibaum.com.